# IGNORE YOUR TEETH and THEY'LL GO AWAY

## THE COMPLETE GUIDE TO GUM DISEASE

Sheldon D. Sydney, D.D.S.

**DEVIDA PUBLICATIONS**

*To*
*Deborah, David, Aviva,*
*Michal and Guy*

DISCLAIMER

This book is a general reference and information guide only, designed to help the reader make informed decisions regarding periodontal health and dental implants. It is not intended as a treatment manual or advice for a particular individual's oral and periodontal problems. Prior to undertaking any treatment including those subjects either discussed or suggested in this book, the reader should seek consultation with a periodontal specialist or experienced dentist trained in the diagnosis and treatment of periodontal disease and dental implants.

Library of Congress Catalogue Card Number 98-93191
ISBN 0-9607498-2-9
Copyright © 1982, 1986 2nd Edition, 1998 3rd Edition
by Sheldon Dov Sydney, D.D.S.

10  9  8  7  6  5  4  3

Printed in the United States of America

**DEVIDA PUBLICATIONS**
205 John Eager Court
Pikesville, Maryland 21208

## Note to the Reader

### What's in a Name... Gum or Periodontal Disease?

When using the expression "gum disease" people are actually referring to a type of periodontal disease, derived from the Latin "peri" for around and "odont" for tooth. "Periodontal" accurately identifies the location of those diseases and conditions affecting the structures immediately surrounding and supporting the teeth (in contrast to dental decay that attacks the teeth themselves). The term "periodontal disease" is used in every major dental text and in communications between health professionals.

However....since the familiar signs of periodontal disease appear in the gums, the expression "gum (which is a lot easier to say than periodontal) disease" has become the lay public's widely preferred and recognized name; it was subsequently selected as the subtitle of this book. In order however, to integrate readers' familiarity with correct terminology, both "gum disease" and "periodontal disease" are used by the author to identify the same disease entities.

# CONTENTS

# IGNORE YOUR TEETH
# and THEY'LL GO AWAY

*The <u>Complete</u> Guide to Gum Disease*

# ACKNOWLEDGEMENTS

My late father and mentor, Dr. Elmer Sydney, my mother Mrs. Fern Sydney Swerdlin, and my wife Rachel, each in their own unique way; and what now seems to have been at the most propitious times, have fortified me with their love, encouragement and unwavering support.

Colleagues, who by association and example have significantly influenced my dental career: Dr. Gerald Bowers, Executive Secretary-Treasurer American Board of Periodontology; Dr John Bergquist, Co-Chair American Board of Periodontology; Dr. Michael Fritz, Charles Howard Candler Professor, Emory University; Dr. Melvin Kushner, Past President, Maryland State Board of Dental Examiners; Dr. Michael McGuire, Vice President, American Academy of Periodontology; Dr. David Noble and Dr. Edward Zwig, private practice of periodontics, Atlanta, Georgia. And my students, on both sides of the Atlantic, who justly persevere in questioning our most cherished beliefs in periodontics, thereby raising the bar of knowledge for all of us in the speciality.

Devida Publications staff especially: executive management team, Sarita and Dan Sragow and marketing director Sharan Kushner, for their consistent attention to the needs of an ever expanding and ambitious project.

Last but certainly not least, my patients; who, for more than twenty years, have never failed to provide me with the inspiration, challenge and fulfillment to work in this wonderful profession.

# INTRODUCTION

## *To the Third Edition*

This updated edition of *Ignore Your Teeth and They'll Go Away* reflects the desire to meet two major goals. Firstly, to maintain the original emphasis of this guide by providing authoritative, comprehensive information with which the consumer can make informed decisions regarding the care of his or her gums. And secondly, to disseminate the significant progress and new techniques that have emerged since the last edition, which have enhanced the periodontist's ability to identify and predictably treat gum diseases.

The reader can be assured that all the procedures and therapies discussed in this guide have been scrupulously evaluated. They are established, predictable treatments based on firm scientific principles. They represent a consensus of the profession as reported in respected publications and supported by peer-reviewed, documented research. Alternative or experimental approaches, when discussed, are clearly identified as such.

Despite the availability of successful periodontal treatments, 80% of all Americans are still affected with gum disease and 44% have already lost all their teeth by the age of 65. But the most alarming of all statistics is that more than half of all school-aged children have gingvitis, the first stage of periodontal disease.

The solution is in your hands. As an informed consumer-patient, you can save your own and your family's teeth from the ravages of gum disease. To begin with, if you have any of the warning signs of gum disease (see page 27) seek immediate professional advice from your dentist or periodontist, an expert in the diagnosis and treatment of gum disease. If you are symptom-free, ask your dentist for a periodontal evaluation during regular check-ups to insure no disease is present. In addition, make use of this book to learn as much as possible about gum disease. Discover how it gets started, diagnosed and treated. Find out why some individuals are more susceptible than others and get the answers to your most commonly asked questions. But most importantly, take to heart the chapter on prevention; there you will acquire the basic techniques of controlling the cause of gum disease...bacterial plaque.

Ignore your teeth and they'll go away? Sure, it's funny, but unfortunately, it's also true! Reading this book, means you have already decided that the health of your gums and teeth is no laughing matter. And that's a good start. Because the more you understand about gum disease, the better are your chances of keeping your teeth for a lifetime of healthy, beautiful smiles.

*Sheldon Dov Sydney*

# PART I

---

*Basic Understandings*

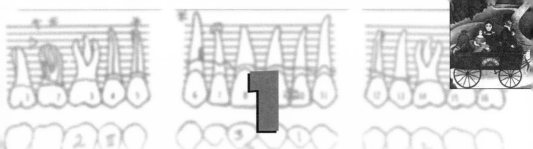

# A JOURNEY BACK IN TIME

## *How History has Recorded Man's Eternal Battle with Gum Disorders*

### DISCOVERIES FROM ANCIENT CIVILIZATIONS

Studies of preserved skulls have established that periodontal (gum) diseases existed in prehistoric times. Recorded history has documented a surprising awareness of periodontal disease throughout the ages.

Embalmed Egyptian mummies from four thousand years ago reveal that periodontal disease was common among the Pharaohs. Ancient papyri also contain significant references to gum problems and suggestions for treatment.

The Sumerians (3000 BC) attempted to practice dental hygiene. Excavations in Mesopotamia have discovered exquisitely designed golden toothpicks used for removing food deposits between the teeth. Later in history, a clay tablet found from the Babylonian and Assyrian periods, revealed that these people suffered from periodontal disease. The clay tablet tells of the need to treat gum problems with massage combined with herbal medicine.

In 2500 BC, Hwang-Fi wrote the oldest known Chinese medical work which included extensive discussion of oral diseases. He divided them into three types: inflammation, diseases of soft tissues of the teeth and tooth decay. He called these three divisions Fong Ya, Ya Kon and Chong Ya, respectively. His work includes accurate descriptions of gum inflammations, abscesses and ulcerations which would be perfectly recognizable today. He describes one condition in this way: "The gingivae are pale or violet red, hard and lumpy, sometimes bleeding, and the toothache is continuous."

The early Hebrews recognized the importance of oral hygiene. Many conditions of the teeth and gums are described in Talmudic writings. A specimen from the ancient Phoenician civilization shows an attempt at wire splinting to stabilize teeth loosened by periodontal disease (Fig. 1-1).

As early as the time of Hippocrates (460-335 BC) it was known that inflammation of the gums could be caused by accumulations of tartar or calculus and that bleeding gums frequently occurred in advanced cases of periodontal disease.

**Fig. 1-1**
A jawbone, excavated from ancient Sidon (1000 BC), demonstrates an early tooth replacement technique. The wire-bound incisors originated in another person's mouth.

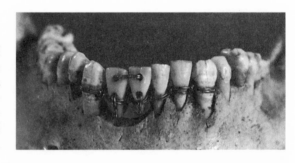

In the first century, the Roman Lulus Cornelius Celsus wrote about diseases affecting the soft tissues of the mouth. He prescribed: "If the gums separate from the teeth, it is beneficial to chew unripe pears and apples and keep their juices in the mouth." He also described teeth loosened by deterioration of the gums, and recommended treating them by touching the gums lightly with a red-hot iron, and then rubbing them with honey and/or narcotics.

Other ancient writers suggested medications ranging from opium, oil of roses and honey, to astringent mouth washes, dentifrice powders, and even counterirritants in treating gum disease. Avicenna (980-1037 BC) was probably the earliest scientist to explore the importance of a proper bite in periodontal disease. He wrote

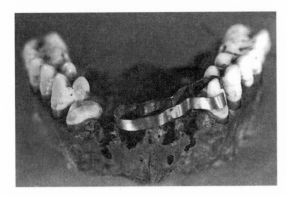

**Fig. 1-2**
The missing front teeth in this Etruscan lower jaw (700 BC) were lost due to severe periodontal disease. The metal band still attached to the canine tooth was part of an attempt to support the teeth which probably became very loose prior to falling out.

about filing elongated teeth to adjust the bite.

About the same time, Albucasis (936-1013 BC) analyzed the need to care for the tooth-supporting structures, and recognized the importance of removing tartar. With a little modernization of language, his writings might be found in a twentieth-century dental text. He wrote: "Sometimes on the surface of the teeth, both inside and outside, as well as under the gums, are deposited rough scales of ugly appearance and black, green or yellow in color. This corruption is communicated to the gums, and so the teeth are, in the process of time, denuded. It is necessary for thee to lay the patient's head upon thy lap and to scrape the teeth and molars, on which are observed either true incrustations, or something similar to sand, and this until nothing more remains of such substance..."

## Perilous Sea Travels

As civilization advanced, man began to travel. Sailors often suffered from extreme vitamin deficiency due to the long and sometimes miscalculated trips between shores. As a result, they developed gum-related Vitamin C deficiency known as *scurvy*, the occupational disease of the time. Lost at sea, many times without supplies and lacking preservatives, the sailors hunted and killed rats for food.

Scurvy, like gum disease, revealed its most devastating effects in the jawbone, loosening teeth and causing severe overgrowth of bleeding gums. In great pain, the sailors would slash each other's gums in order to reduce the pressure from this uncontrollable infection.

## NAMES WORTH REMEMBERING

When Anton van Leevuenhoek (1632-1723) invented the microscope, he was certainly unaware that over two hundred years later, the little creatures he found and described through his lens (taken from the saliva of his own mouth) would become the bacterial foundation for the study of periodontal disease. What he saw then for the first time were plaque-forming germs or bacteria!

It was with his book published in 1728, "The Surgeon Dentist – a Treatise on Teeth," that Pierre Fauchard (Fig. 1-3) emerged as the father of modern dentistry. The Frenchman wrote on a broad range of

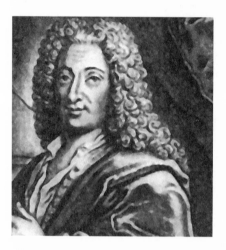

**Fig. 1-3**
Pierre Fauchard had a prolific professional and social life (he married three times). One of his less illustrious suggestions however was the transplanting of teeth to replace missing teeth. The idea caught on, and for a time, a premium price was paid by dentists to those willing to sell their natural teeth to be transplanted into someone else's jaw. In fact, Victor Hugo's *Les Miserables*, of the early 1800's tells of the selling of Fantine's two extracted incisors for forty francs.

dental subjects from dental chairs to dentures. In particular, his writings on *pyorrhea* (an old name for gum disease) were so often quoted that for a time it was called "Fauchard's Disease."

England's John Hunter, a physician and surgeon, expanded current knowledge of teeth and gums with his work "The Natural History of the Human Teeth" published in 1778. In this now classic text, Hunter accurately described how gum disease began at the gum edge, working its way down the root and eventually destroying the connection of the tooth to the bone.

In the United States, Dr. John M. Riggs (1810-1885) of Hartford, Connecticut probably did more than any other individual to establish the basis of modern periodontics with his use of specific instruments

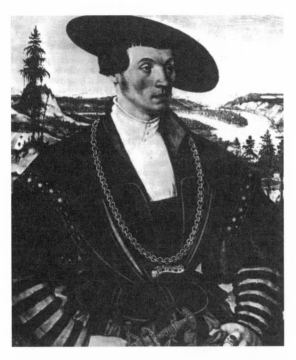

**Fig. 1-4**
This painting by Hans von Shonitz depicts a well dressed Italian nobleman around 1500. Being perfectly attired, included wearing a neck chain holding an exquisitely designed case containing soft gold toothpicks (which he proudly displayed after meals!)

in the successful treatment of gum disease. He was a frequent lecturer and author who encouraged many dentists to adopt his methods. Though he originally began his education as a priest and later attended medical school, Dr. Riggs eventually chose dentistry and specifi-

## DR. RIGGS' SPECIAL PLACE IN HISTORY

Dr. John Riggs was a participant in one of the most dramatic advances in medicine. His colleague and friend Dr. Horace Wells, who discovered anesthesia, once saw a circus show where "laughing gas" or nitrous oxide was being demonstrated. Being inquisitive and also suffering from a toothache too advanced for Dr. Riggs' methods, Dr. Wells asked that Riggs remove the tooth after administering the gas. This having been done with no pain, gave Riggs the distinction of having performed the first surgical procedure with the aid of anesthesia.

cally periodontics as a career. Some of his basic techniques still have applications in today's modern therapy.

# DENTAL EDUCATION

Early on, dentistry was taught as an apprenticeship because no formal dental colleges existed. Chapin Harris, a physician, became interested in dentistry and traveled throughout the southern United States

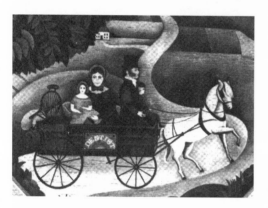

**Fig. 1-5**
The early days of dental practice in the United States found the dentist traveling with his family and equipment from town to town to deliver needed dental care. The sign on the wagon reads "Dentist."

practicing dentistry and medicine. He moved to Baltimore and studied with Horace Hayden, a dentist who lectured to medical students at the University of Baltimore.

Harris and Hayden hoped to develop a department of dentistry in the university's medical school, but were unable to gain acceptance by the faculty. They petitioned the State of Maryland for a charter and in 1840 the Baltimore College of Dental Surgery became the first dental college in the world with the authority to award a D.D.S. (Doctor of Dental Surgery). Dr. F. H. Rehwinkel a German physician became interested in dentistry and graduated from the Maryland dental school in 1854. He is credited with first using the term "pyorrhea" to describe gum disease in a paper presented in August, 1877.

## The Speciality of Periodontics

Soon the need developed for formalized, advanced education beyond the basic dental degree, for dentists who could provide specialized skills to patients suffering from diseases of the gums and tooth-supporting structures. The speciality that emerged to meet this need would be known as *periodontics*, and the specialist in these diseases, a *periodontist*. In 1914, The American Academy of Periodontology (AAP) was founded. Over the ensuing years, the Academy has done much to advance the periodontal health of the public and promote excellence in the practice of periodontics. This includes the establishment and continuing quality assurance of specialty programs in periodontics throughout the country.

Today, the AAP is the principal authority on all matters dealing with periodontics for health care providers and consumers. In addition, the AAP represents dental professionals specializing in the prevention, diagnosis and treatment of periodontal diseases, and the placement and treatment of dental implants.

Dramatic advances continue to be made by dedicated researchers and clinicians in our understanding of gum diseases, leading to an ever increasing range of predictable therapies. However, it should be clear by now, that today's discoveries have not developed in a vacuum, but are built on the shoulders of giants from a remarkable history.

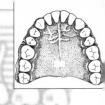

# 2

# THE JAWBONE'S CONNECTED TO THE...

## A Close-Up Look at the Anatomy of a Healthy Mouth

### THE TEETH AND THEIR SUPPORTING MECHANISM

E ach tooth is unique in size, shape and function. *Molars*, for example, have large, wide–biting surfaces and two or three roots that are utilized for the heavy biting pressures necessary to emulsify the food. *Incisors*, on the other hand, are shaped for their shearing ability, because they tear the food into smaller pieces for the molars to chew.

Teeth grow out of sockets formed from the upper and lower jawbones called *alveolar bone,* which surround the roots of the teeth and provide support during chewing.

The tooth, however, does not fit exactly within the socket. A slight space between tooth and bone contains fibrous threads of tissue that hold the tooth to the bone and provide a shock-absorbing layer permitting slight movement under pressure. These highly specialized fiber attachments are called the *periodontal ligaments*. Alongside the periodontal ligaments, pass blood vessels that act as conduits for nutrition and nerves that carry signals from the brain. The signals transfer information relative to the exact position of the teeth and

**Fig. 2-1**

# THE TEETH

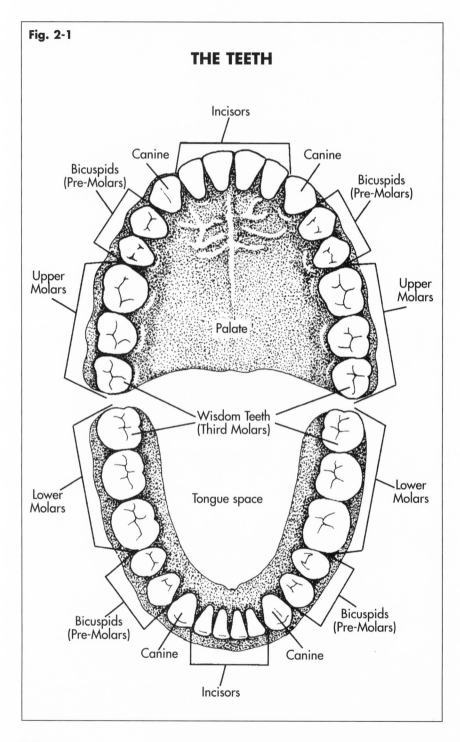

Incisors

Canine

Canine

Bicuspids
(Pre-Molars)

Bicuspids
(Pre-Molars)

Upper
Molars

Upper
Molars

Palate

Wisdom Teeth
(Third Molars)

Lower
Molars

Lower
Molars

Tongue space

Bicuspids
(Pre-Molars)

Bicuspids
(Pre-Molars)

Canine

Canine

Incisors

jaws, from the brain to the tongue and cheek during chewing and speech.

Periodontal ligaments are embedded in a special root surface called the *cementum*. The cementum has a porous surface that facilitates adherence to the periodontal ligament.

Finally, the *enamel* is the hard, protective outer layer covering the exposed portion of the tooth above the gum line, and the first defense against cavities.

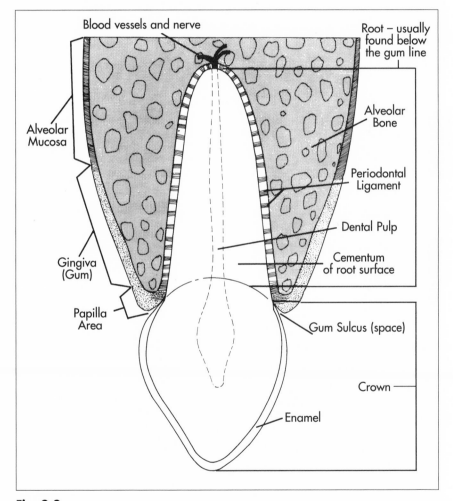

**Fig. 2-2**
The tooth, gum and supporting bone, as seen in a cross-section view of an upper tooth.

Inside the body of the tooth is found the *dental pulp*. Within it are the nerves, blood vessels and other life-supporting mechanisms that keep the interior of the tooth healthy.

# THE GUMS (GINGIVA)

Several different tissues comprise what we know as "gums." The technical name is *gingiva* and includes the tissues that extend from the jaws to the necks of the teeth.

The gingiva is the coral-pink tissue which blankets the area of the root and bone, providing important protection for these underlying structures. The triangular shaped *papilla* is an extension of the gingiva which fills the space between the teeth (Fig. 2-3).

Around the neck of each tooth, the gingiva has a fold of tissue that forms a small v-shaped groove called the *sulcus*. The sulcus is where most periodontal disease starts. Usually the gum sulcus is slightly over a millimeter or two in depth, or about one tenth of an inch. Under

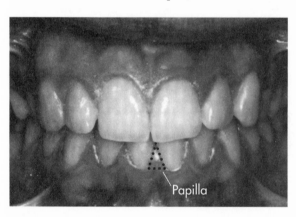

Papilla

**Fig. 2-3**
A healthy smile reveals well defined gum lines that form the triangular papilla between the teeth.

healthy conditions, the sulcus is tightly adapted to the tooth and free of contaminants.

Continuing past the gingiva into the furrow where the lip and jawbone meet, is the *alveolar mucosa*. This thin, almost transparent tissue is a direct continuation of the gingiva, although technically not gingiva. The alveolar mucosa which covers the jawbone (alveolar bone) has a glistening appearance which usually contrasts sharply with the leathery and pale texture of the gingiva.

# 3

# PERIODONTAL DISEASES

## *How We Progress from a Normal Tooth to Toothless Gums*

Despite these warning signs, periodontal disease affects nearly 75% of all adults. How this disease can work so insidiously and destructively is a subject worthy of further understanding.

# BACTERIAL PLAQUE

Without question, the number one cause of periodontal or gum disease is *bacterial plaque*. Plaque is a thin, colorless, sticky substance found on tooth surfaces.

How is plaque formed? Within a few minutes after a tooth has been completely cleaned, the process of plaque formation begins. Bacteria in the mouth begin collecting either directly on the surface of the teeth

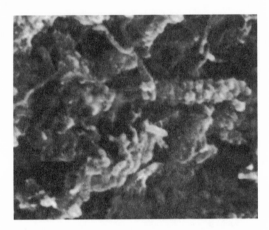

**Fig. 3-1**
This microscopic view of plaque shows a number of gum disease-causing germs. Over 500 specific bacteria have been identified to be in the human mouth at any particular time. Those that are more virulent and invasive wreak the greatest damage on the gums and tooth-supporting bone.
Photograph courtesy of Dr. Jon Suzuki.

or on the *pellicle* which is an intervening, imperceptible coating formed on the teeth from proteins in the saliva.

Additional layers of deposits and bacteria adhere to and expand the plaque surface, so that within hours after teeth have been thoroughly cleaned, measurable amounts of plaque can be detected (Fig. 3-1). The rate of plaque accumulation varies in different individuals and on different teeth in a particular person.

Left completely alone with no effort to remove it, plaque will reach a maximum thickness of a soft white material in about thirty days. During the course of the build-up, the bacteria become more virulent. If allowed to continue unabated, plaque bacteria will release poisons or toxins that stimulate the destructive series of events leading to gum disease.

## Calculus (Tartar)

Traces of mineral salts found in saliva combine with the plaque to form a hard, porous, calcified deposit on the teeth called *calculus*, more commonly known as *tartar*. Chemically speaking, calculus is a cousin of boiler scale, and is no more desirable in your mouth than clogged pipes in your home, as it provides an attractive surface for plaque accumulation.

## THE BATTLE FOR SUPERIORITY – How we react to plaque

When you catch a cold, it is not actually the invading cold virus that causes you to have the fever, headaches, sniffles and sneezing. Those symptoms are all part of the body's response to the invading virus. Our understanding of this phenomenon comes by way of the study of microbiology (germs) and immunology (the human defensive systems). The battle between the invading bacterial plaque and the defense devices of one's own body is central to understanding the destructive results of periodontal disease.

When gum tissue cells recognize that they are in contact with potentially destructive bacterial plaque or its poisons, the body's protective system sends out blood, rich in defensive equipment, to fight the invaders. The battle goes on as the bacteria attempt to gain superiority in numbers and strength, while the immune system fights back vigorously with its own defensive mechanisms. The battle can lead to red and swollen gum tissue and the beginning of a destructive disease cycle.

### Host Response

Today, the term *host response* is used to describe the unique nature of each human or host to mount an effective defense to infection. Regarding periodontal disease, we have discovered many aspects of the host response that influence an individual's reaction to plaque and its toxins.

Unfortunately, there is still much we do not understand. In the future, this ever expanding field is likely to provide us with new basic tools with which to treat or prevent disease. For now, we can summarize this subject by saying that if an individual has a good host response, the damaged caused by the gum diseases will likely be less destructive than in an individual with a poor host response.

# GINGIVITIS

*Gingivitis,* an early gum infection, is a reversible disease characterized by tenderness, swelling, and most importantly, bleeding of the gum tissue. In the United States, a majority of youngsters over the age of thirteen already have gingivitis! The normal, healthy pink color darkens from the increase in blood volume, and goes through various

## BLEEDING GUMS – IS ANYONE PAYING ATTENTION?

How is it so many esthetic–minded, health conscious, intelligent people allow their gums to bleed day in and day out without the slightest concern? Why is there so little anxiety about gum bleeding? Bleeding indicates that there is an infection present, thus warning of danger to the gums, just as infection would be a serious concern elsewhere in the body. There is no question that blood oozing from the ear or coughed-up would send most of us running immediately to a professional for help. Why? Because we know bleeding always signifies something is wrong! Bleeding in the mouth however has been considered "normal" for so long that this important early warning sign is being ignored (remember the title of this book?). Any amount of bleeding in the mouth must be evaluated by a periodontist or other dental professional.

shades of red. In more advanced cases, the gums may appear reddish-blue. Gingivitis usually begins gradually and progresses as symptoms become more prominent. It can, however, be a fluctuating disease. For example, inflamed areas develop and then become normal, only for inflammation to reappear at a later date.

# THE PERIODONTAL POCKET

If plaque accumulation did no more than cause irritation or gingivitis, we might not be so concerned. Unfortunately, because most bleeding is ignored, the advantage is lost of detecting early signs of periodontal disease and receiving prompt and relatively simple care. If the disease progresses, serious consequences can develop.

As noted earlier, the gum reacts to plaque with swelling and inflammation. This condition permits the plaque to approach the normally well-adapted crevice or sulcus between the gingiva and tooth. The infection spreads down into the attachment causing the gum to separate from the tooth.

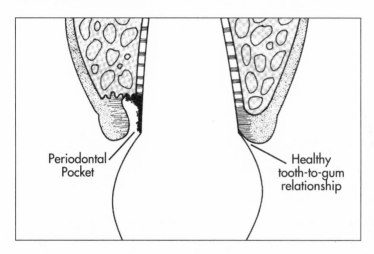

Periodontal Pocket

Healthy tooth-to-gum relationship

**Fig. 3-2**
Periodontal Pocket

With the gum seal broken, more plaque can bury itself within the newly enlarged gum space. The space created by this separation is called a *periodontal pocket* (Fig. 3-2) and represents the critical pathologic entity of periodontal disease. In general, it is the comparative measurement of these pockets that reveals the extent and seriousness of periodontal disease.

## PERIODONTITIS

As the gum infection advances along the root, the pocket deepens with destruction of bone and attaching fibers. This condition, typically found in adults, is called *periodontitis* or more specifically *adult periodontitis*, and is the most common periodontal disease affecting the tooth-supporting bone. The disease is also distinguished by its severity, i.e. early, moderate or advanced periodontitis.

31

**Fig. 3-3**

# PROGRESS OF PERIODONTAL DISEASE

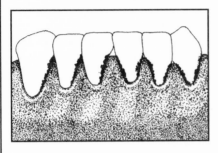

### GINGIVITIS

Plaque and tartar accumulate along the gum lines and the necks of the teeth. Gums swell and begin to show evidence of bleeding. Gums are no longer well adapted to the tooth and the gum space (sulcus) may be open.

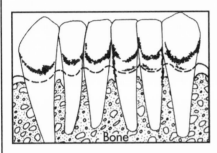

### EARLY TO MODERATE PERIODONTITIS

(gum tissues not drawn in)

Plaque advances below the gum line along with the begining of pocket formation. Early bone loss is noted which may be accompanied by recession of the gums (dotted line).

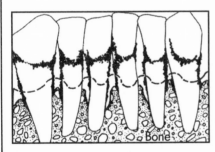

### ADVANCED PERIODONTITIS

Teeth are loose as plaque and tartar advance down the root surfaces.

The gum line may continue to recede.

Bone is destroyed leaving deep defects and pockets filled with infection.

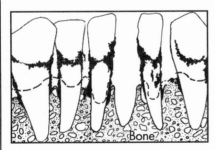

### SEVERE PERIODONTITIS AND TOOTH LOSS

Serious infection is present.

Very loose teeth, pus and abscess formation are likely to occur along with the loss of teeth.

Periodontitis has been referred to as pyorrhea, which literally means "pus flow." Pus can develop as supporting bone is destroyed and interacts with the infected gum tissue, usually in the latter stages of the disease. Sometimes so much support is destroyed that the teeth become loose. Periodontitis is serious business. When left untreated, periodontitis has the potential to continue in adulthood for many years as a chronic, progressive infection, and a true threat to the life of the teeth (Fig. 3-3).

## EARLY ONSET PERIODONTITIS – Children and Young Adults

A group of periodontal diseases far less common than adult periodontitis is known as *early onset periodontitis* (EOP). Individuals with EOP demonstrate significant bone loss around their teeth at a young age (some as early as 4-5 years old). This bone loss is not always proportional to the amount of plaque found in the mouth.

*Juvenile periodontitis,* the most frequently observed form of EOP, may first appear around the time of puberty. This disease can involve a few isolated teeth or the entire mouth. The local type seems to be somewhat self-limiting, while the general form is often more aggressive and progressive. The term *rapidly progressive periodontitis* is sometimes applied to individuals in their early twenties to mid-thirties, who demonstrate the characteristics of the generalized form of juvenile periodontitis.

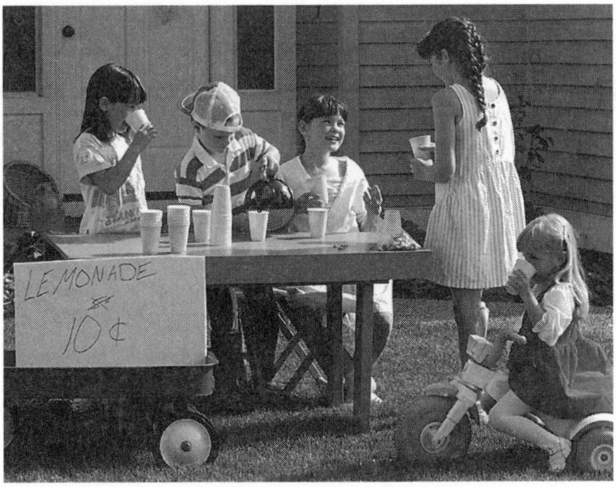

**Fig. 3-4**
Though generally thought of as an adult problem, the EOP form of periodontal disease can affect even young children.

33

EOP patients do not always respond to routine therapy. Systemic diseases are known to be associated with certain forms of EOP. Studies have indicated that EOP may be influenced by defective cells in the body's defense mechanism. Also, as it often appears among family members, a genetic predisposition to EOP has been hypothesized.

## REFRACTORY PERIODONTITIS

*Refractory periodontitis* is a recurring form of periodontal disease which has been resistant or not responsive to established methods of treatment. Smoking and underlying systemic conditions have been suggested as being associated with the disease.

## RECESSION-EXPOSED ROOTS

Occasionally gum tissues recede along with the loss of bone, especially on the front root surfaces of the teeth where the bone is thin and the roots tend to bulge. Often accompanying the esthetic defect is temperature sensitivity resulting from root exposure. Some recession is caused by heavy tooth brushing. A hard scrubbing technique can lead to recession without inflammation being present.

**Fig. 3-5**
Typical appearance of recession and exposed roots is seen in these lower incisors.

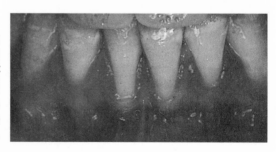

## TRENCH MOUTH

*Acute necrotizing ulcerative gingivitis* (ANUG) or its more popular term *trench mouth* is characterized by a painful gum infection that can last as long as several weeks. This disease is a unique, sometimes recurring condition which can develop independently of gingivitis, but can nonetheless lead to bone loss.

The widespread prevalence of ANUG among World War I soldiers gave rise to the "trench mouth" name. The condition however was even recognized in the fourth century during the Greek Empire. Xenophon described that fighters of the time were affected by "sore mouths" and foul-smelling breath. Later in the 19th century, reports of an epidemic of this disease in the French army found their way into historical literature.

Though long considered to be contagious, more recent research has proved that this is not the case. The latest studies suggest that in addition to plaque – stress, smoking and poor nutrition are often associated with the disease.

# SPECIAL GUM PROBLEMS

## Common But Less Well-known Ailments

M any conditions affect the gums which are not strictly members of the gingivitis or periodontitis family. Reviewed in this chapter are some of the more common special gum problems one might encounter.

### PRIMARY ORAL HERPES

One of the few confirmed contagious gum diseases is *primary oral herpes* or *acute herpetic gingivostomatitis.* It generally lasts from a week to ten days. Frequently seen in children, it is caused by a virus. Symptoms include painful white and red sores in the gum area that may spread to the lips and throat. This disease is generally associated with a fever. Primary herpes is not the same virus that causes genital herpes which results from sexual contact.

### ABSCESS (GUM BOIL)

An *abscess* (gum boil) is a collection of infected gum and sometimes bone tissue resulting in the formation of pus. It can cause pain. These isolated lesions usually develop from infection underneath the gum tissue within pre-existing periodontal pockets. Abscesses may also occur in healthy gums as a result of trapped food or foreign matter such as broken toothpicks.

## CANKER SORES

Small, white ulcerated areas found on the inside of the lips and mouth are usually *canker sores* or *apthous ulcers.* They are generally painful, especially when eating spicy foods, and last about ten days. While the cause has not been determined conclusively, some hypotheses include stress, nutritional or vitamin deficiency and allergy. Anesthetic creams placed directly on the sores are generally helpful until the symptoms subside.

## INJURIES TO GUM TISSUE

Many instances of accidental injury to the gum tissues have been reported in dental literature. Cuts in the gums are caused by uninten-

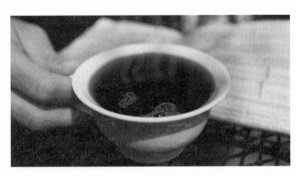

**Fig. 4-1**
Hot beverages can contribute to accidental injury of the mouth's sensitive tissues.

tional scratching with fingernails as well as the improper use of dental floss, toothpicks and hard toothbrushes. The unjustified custom of placing aspirin tablets directly on painful gums has lead to serious chemical burns. Also scalding soups and drinks, pizza or other hot foods can leave a very sore blister on the roof of the mouth.

## CHANGES IN GUM COLOR

A change in gum color can result from the absorption of certain heavy metals. Arsenic and mercury, for example, can produce a black line that follows the shape of the gum margin. Lead in the blood results in a bluish-red or deep purple line along the gum margin, while silver produces a bluish-gray discoloration throughout the membranes of the mouth. Medicines such as minocycline, frequently used in acne therapy, are known to produce a black appearance to the gums. Alteration in gum color may also be caused by underlying medical problems. Addison's disease, for example, which is signified by a deficiency in a specialized hormone, may produce isolated black or brown patches on the gums.

## PUFFY GUMS

Puffy or swollen gums may be caused by conditions other than gum disease. Drugs used to prevent seizures, and certain heart medications, for example, can cause the gums to become puffy. Some forms of anemia and leukemia also produce distinctive enlargement of the gum tissue.

## PERICORONITIS

*Pericoronitis* is a relatively common occurrence usually resulting when gum tissue grows over wisdom teeth (especially those that are not fully erupted) and become swollen and painful. This condition is exacerbated by biting on the swollen gums. Treatment involves either removal of the tooth, or treatment of the affected gum.

## SKIN DISEASES

There are various skin diseases that also affect the soft tissues of the mouth. Some involve a local response to a specific allergy, while others can represent a generalized skin problem with complicating oral symptoms, such as psoriasis. A periodontist is trained to recognize these diseases and will in many cases, work with a skin specialist (dermatologist) to treat the problem.

## GROWTHS

Tumors or growths, both benign and malignant (cancerous), occur in the mouth and gum tissues. A trained professional is the only one who can evaluate if a growth is serious or not. A sample or biopsy of the suspected lesion may be required to confirm the diagnosis.

# PART II

*Evaluation*

# 5

# A VISIT TO THE PERIODONTIST

## *What to Expect*

Most patients are referred for consultation by their dentists, friends or physicians. This is the moment when they may hear the word "periodontist" for the first time, and are confronted with the possibility that they have a disease requiring attention by a specialist.

The fact that periodontal disease does not usually cause pain, further mystifies the patient who generally associates disease with discomfort or other annoying symptoms. Along with this natural concern is a phenomenon of great anticipation resulting from second-hand "gum treatment experiences," related to the patient as soon as periodontal disease is brought up in casual conversation.

### Who is this Stranger, the Periodontist?

To begin with, all dentists go through the same basic preparatory training. First they obtain an undergraduate degree from college or university. This is followed by four years of dental school, whereupon a dentist will receive either a D.D.S. (Doctor of Dental Surgery), or a D.M.D. (Doctor of Dental Medicine). Both of these degrees are identical in regard to the type of education and qualifications as a dentist.

A qualified dentist, if accepted, then attends an approved specialty program which requires an additional three years of training, principally in the study of periodontal disease and dental implants. The competition for acceptance into these programs is keen. During their extensive training, periodontists become proficient in the latest techniques and advances in diagnosis and treatment. Following the successful completion of the specialty program, the periodontist receives a postdoctoral certificate and becomes eligible for active membership into the American Academy of Periodontology (AAP). Individuals qualified to announce themselves as *Specialists in Periodontics* include active AAP members and limit their practices to the treatment of periodontal diseases, and the placement and maintenance of dental implants.

## THE MEDICAL HISTORY

Using a detailed questionnaire as a guide, the periodontist will ask about your general health. He or she will be interested to know about your diet, smoking history, current medications, allergies and sensitivities to drugs. Recent changes in your general health will be of special importance. If you have a history of heart disease, lung disease, diabetes, nerve disorders, psychological problems or tumors, the periodontist will want to confer with your physician to see how this information could influence the course of your disease and its treatment. Your medical condition may even be influenced by the presence of periodontal disease (see opposite page).

## THE DENTAL HISTORY

This part of the discussion usually includes questions such as: When was the patient first told or recognized that gum disease was present? Has there been any treatment? What plaque control methods are in current use? Does the patient understand the importance of daily plaque removal? This last question is pertinent to the successful treatment of periodontal disease. Patients need to be aware that their motivation and participation are key factors. There will also be many questions relating to current and previous dental care. What brought

44

## THE INFLUENCE OF PERIODONTAL DISEASE ON MEDICAL CONDITIONS

The relationship between periodontal disease and medical conditions or diseases has generated both great interest and concern. There is increasing evidence suggesting that the presence of advanced periodontal disease can influence the initiation and/or the course of certain medical problems. Some of the most recent developments in this area include the following:

- Reports appearing both in the professional and lay press have implicated that the presence of advanced periodontal disease may lead to the birth of premature <u>low birth-weight babies.</u>

- In studies performed in the U.S. and Scandinavia, <u>heart disease</u> was found to be more frequent in patients with advanced periodontal disease.

- A similar investigation reported an increased likelihood of <u>stroke</u> and <u>subsequent death</u> for patients with advanced periodontal disease.

- As far back as 1960, an article published in a leading national journal suggested that the control of periodontal infection reduced the need for insulin in <u>diabetic patients.</u> Today, the American Diabetes Association recognizes periodontal disease as a significant consideration in the care of diabetes.

One of the hypotheses suggested to explain these findings is that the gum disease-causing bacteria, its toxins and/or the accumulation of other elements in the defense system extend their influence beyond the locally infected site, allowing areas far removed from the mouth to become endangered. At this point in our understanding, prudent advice would be to encourage everyone with the noted medical conditions to be evaluated for the presence of periodontal disease.

you to the dentist previously? Do you have any special concerns about your mouth, such as esthetics?

# HEAD AND FACE EXAM

After completing the history, attention is given to the exterior of the head, face and neck, looking for any abnormalities in shape or size. This examination is important in revealing swelling, changes in skin texture or coloration, and will include palpation of the glands in the neck.

## The TM Joint

The *TM joint* or TMJ (*temporomandibular joint*) is a part of the jaw located in front of the ear that acts as a hinge (Fig. 5-1). To find the TMJ, place your fingers just in front of your ear around where the temples are located; you will feel the movement of these joints as you open and close your jaws. Damage to the TMJ and its associated muscles, which can result from accidents and bite problems, are termed

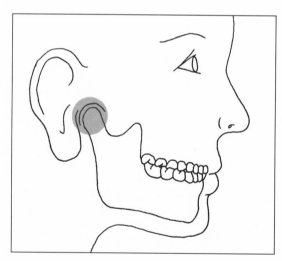

**Fig. 5-1**
The TM joint (shaded area) is composed of the uppermost extension of the lower jawbone and an indentation on the upper jaw. Along with a series of muscles, the TM Joint controls all movement of the lower jaw.

*TM disorders.* The symptoms of TM disorders include popping, cracking or clicking in the area of the ear, a history of soreness in the jaw, and severe wear of the teeth. It has been noted that patients with TM disorders may also suffer from headaches, dizziness, neck and shoulder pains.

# THE PERIODONTAL EXAMINATION

A detailed look into the mouth is next. Identifying the amount of plaque and calculus that is present is necessary. Gum color, consistency, type, quantity and quality, and level of inflammation will be noted. The periodontist will be interested in knowing if teeth are sensitive during eating, brushing, or as a result of instrument contact. Areas of food impaction, teeth that are rotated or otherwise out of normal position will be recorded. A careful observation will be made of missing teeth, as well as the quality of various dental treatments you have had to date. Old fillings and crowns will be evaluated to determine if they need repair or replacement.

## Diagnostic Tests

Occasionally the use of one or more tests may be required to assist in establishing a correct diagnosis or in assessing the extent of disease activity. A *biopsy* requires the removal of a small portion of tissue for microscopic examination. It is essential for evaluating suspicious growths. *Blood studies* may be indicated if medical problems are suspected of complicating the periodontal condition.

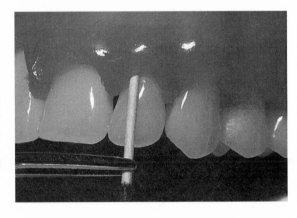

**Fig. 5-2**
A filter tip or strip may be used to remove a small amount of gum fluid for examination.

*Cultures* or other bacteria-identifying examinations can be helpful in developing the precise treatment that will be prescribed for you. Sampling of gum fluids found in the sulcus may indicate the level of disease activity. *Gene analysis* will likely become a more common procedure to identify patients susceptible to advanced gum disease.

47

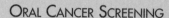

ORAL CANCER SCREENING

Evaluation of the lips, tongue, floor of the mouth, palate, cheeks and throat will be made to check for any signs of oral cancer. Although oral cancer is fortunately not frequently found, an early diagnosis is critical.

## The Periodontal Probe: a Key Investigating Tool

The fundamental tool used in the examination is the *periodontal probe*. This is a miniature ruler, especially designed to measure the gum sulcus or crevice. On its face are notches at calibrated intervals of one or more millimeters apart. The probe is placed between the tooth and gum until some resistance is felt, indicating where the gum is attached to the tooth (Fig.5-3). Normal measurements range up to three millimeters which translates to a maximum of 1/8 inch (the size of a normal sulcus). In general, any measurement above three millimeters may be considered a periodontal pocket; damage can be expected to have already taken place in that area.

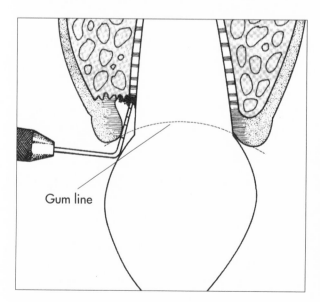

Gum line

**Fig. 5-3**
The periodontal probe measures the distance from the gum line to the bottom of the gum space. Measurements greater than three millimeters are generally considered periodontal pockets.

For example, a five millimeter pocket would generally indicate that some of the tooth-supporting bone has been destroyed. Ten millimeters would suggest that perhaps 80-90% of the bone has been lost.

A complete analysis will include six measurements around each tooth. Remember gum lines run along the front, sides and back of teeth. Two hundred measurements in one mouth is normal, and will give a detailed typographical profile of the mouth (Fig.5-4). You need not worry about the number of measurements. You will hardly notice this procedure. Periodontal probe measurements are often called out by the periodontist and recorded by an assistant.

The otherwise mysterious conversation at this point might sound like "... upper right incisor 5...6...9, upper right molar 5...3...9," and so on in succession until all teeth are recorded. With the completion of this part of the examination, we have a detailed map of all your periodontal pockets.

## PSR®-A Simple Test for Gum Disease

Your dentist may have used a special, colored periodontal probe during a PSR® (Periodontal Screening and Recording™) examination. This simple evaluation system, which is endorsed by the American Academy of Periodontology and the American Dental Association, can detect periodontal disease and result in early diagnosis and treatment.

Briefly, the mouth is divided into six sections. Each section is examined for a number of signs including bleeding and probing depth. Scores range from "0," which suggests no gum disease up to a score of "3" or "4" indicating that a more comprehensive examination is necessary.

## Checking the Bite

The bite or *occlusion* is best described as the relationship of the teeth to each other in normal, closed and chewing positions. The patient is asked to chew, and slide the upper teeth over the lower teeth. Areas where excess pressure is noted will be recorded for later use. Teeth with abnormal wear or movement will also be noted. Plaster molds of the teeth may be made for further study.

## Tooth Movement

Tooth movement or *mobility* is an important sign of excess tooth pressure and/or periodontal disease. Each tooth is tested. The results are transformed into a number system. Again, working in millimeters, the indications of mobility are "one," two," or "three," which signify the degree of movement. "One" is considered early mobility. "Three," which is about 1/8 inch side to side, would be very significant movement. Sometimes patients are unaware of mobile teeth.

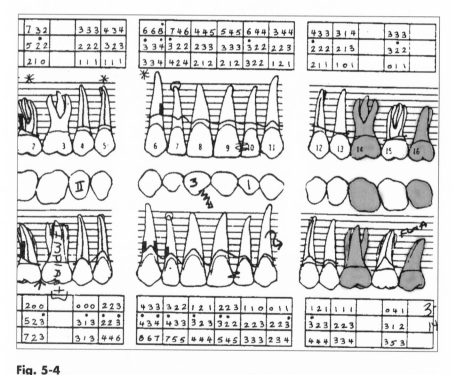

**Fig. 5-4**

The periodontal chart is used to record and calculate probing measurements from various reference points, in addition to other important findings such as tooth mobility, recession and missing teeth. This is an essential document that will be used to plan and monitor the patient's treatment.

# X-RAYS

The examination thus far has involved those areas directly visible to the therapist. The use of *x-rays* or *radiographs* provides essential information by revealing differences in hardness and density in hard and soft tissues. X-rays are generally negative pictures in gray, black, and white. The whiter the image the greater the density. A silver filling or gold cap would appear white because radiation does not easily pass through. The tongue, gums and cheeks appear dark and are not readily discernible.

Radiographs allow the detection of early bone breakdown around teeth as well as the size and shape of roots, cavities, cysts, signs of bite trauma, the need for a possible root canal, extra teeth and bone tumors.

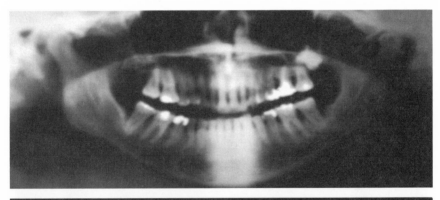

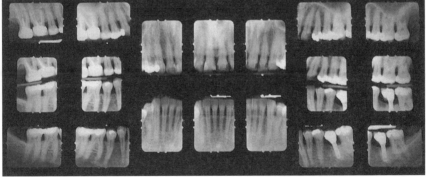

**Fig. 5-5**
The panoramic x-ray (above) gives a general view of the mouth and jaws, while the periapical set (below) shows details of each tooth and its surrounding area.

## Types of X-Rays

Two major applications of x-rays are used (Fig. 5-5). One is the *panoramic* x-ray in which a general view of all the teeth and jaws is shown in one large rectangular view.

A second type, which is preferred in the diagnosis of periodontal disease, is the *periapical* x-ray taken with small squares of film placed against the teeth by a plastic holder. When the films are arranged together in a frame, periapical x-rays give a detailed view of each tooth and its supporting bone. The average complete or full mouth series of periapical x-rays consists of sixteen to twenty individual films.

Additional radiographs may be suggested if dental implants are being considered or if there is need for more precise details of a suspicious area. For example, a *CT scan* (*computerized tomography*) is a computer-based x-ray which reveals specific areas of the jaw in three dimensions.

# 6

# THE PROGNOSIS

## Forecasting a Future for Your Teeth

After completing the evaluation process, the periodontist will meet with the patient to review the information obtained during the examination, the results of any laboratory tests and the x-ray findings. In addition, the patient will be presented with a suggested plan of treatment (more on this in the next chapter), the time involved and the expected fee.

There will be a discussion about the specific nature of his/her periodontal disease. Educational materials will be offered on the subject which not only explain the disease but go a long way in reassuring the patient that he or she is not alone. In fact, many people are comforted to know that they do not have a rare disease.

Once patients understand their periodontal disease and the proposed treatment, it is not uncommon to hear the question "Okay, if I complete the treatment, pay the fee and follow directions, how long will I keep my teeth?"

*Prognosis* is the technique of forecasting the future of your teeth, based on the anticipated course of the disease in conjunction with the opportunity to provide appropriate treatment. Just as the meteorolo-

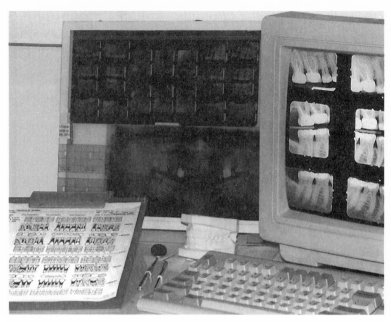

**Fig. 6-1**
All available information is used to develop the treatment plan and prognosis.

gist relies on many sources of data to forecast the weather, so peri-odontists need to harness all their accumulated scientific skills and experience, to establish an accurate and reliable forecast or prognosis of the teeth.

No two patients are exactly alike. Some may appear similar at first but will yield quite different results. This is because periodontal dis-ease is a multi-factorial disease. In other words, although we know that plaque is the primary cause of gum disease, there are other influ-ences that modify the character of the disease and the determination of the prognosis. Sometimes these influences are referred to as *risk factors* or just *factors* because they may place patients at risk for more serious periodontal problems.

The various factors that influence the disease process and progno-sis are identified prior to the start of therapy to assist in establishing a treatment plan suited to the individual patient. For purposes of clari-ty, these factors have been divided into two areas. *General* factors affect the individual as a whole and could also impact on other health problems or conditions. Many of these factors help determine the patient's host response as discussed on page 29.

*Local* factors tend to be limited in their influence and have a more direct effect on the oral structures.

# GENERAL FACTORS INFLUENCING THE PROGNOSIS

## Systemic Diseases

Systemic diseases and/or the medications associated with their treatment may increase the severity of periodontal disease. The more common examples include diabetes, compromised immunity conditions, blood diseases and cardiovascular illness.

## Stress

There are highly suggestive scientific findings which indicate that stress can have a significant effect on the severity of gum disease, as well as an adverse influence on the body's response to treatment.

## Genetic Predisposition

We now have the ability to locate specific genetic factors that predict susceptibility to gum disease. The use of this information and the likelihood of its expanding application have created great promise for identifying patients who are at particular risk for advanced periodontal disease.

## Smoking

Smokers are more likely to build up excessive calculus, unsightly stain and bad breath. Research has confirmed that tobacco use leads to gum recession, mouth sores, deeper periodontal pockets and a

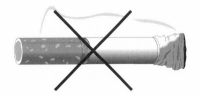

**Fig 6-2**
Smoking is not only bad for your general health, but also has a definite negative effect on the extent and severity of gum disease.

greater chance of loosing one's teeth. The results of therapy will also be compromised. It should be noted that smokeless tobacco can have similar effects, including a significant risk of oral cancer.

## Age

Surprisingly, for two patients with the same amount of disease the prognosis is better for the older patient than for the younger one. The reason is that the older individual has managed to preserve a certain amount of bone for a long period of time. Losing bone slowly, while undesirable, is still the expected course for untreated periodontal disease. The younger patient, having a rapid-type bone loss, suggests that additional influences need to be addressed (see EOP page 33).

## Special Problems for Women

Changes in women's hormonal balance may influence the reaction of gum tissue to plaque and calculus. Women are particularly susceptible to gum problems during puberty, menstruation, pregnancy, menopause and while taking oral contraceptives.

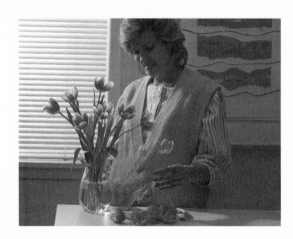

**Fig. 6-3**
Pregnancy can cause an intensified reaction of the gum tissues to plaque, leading to increased inflammation and bleeding.

For example a condition known as a *pregnancy tumor* while not a true tumor describes a growth of gum tissue often seen during pregnancy. This growth is due to a heightened response of the gum tissue to irritation. Also, *osteoporosis*, a common problem from the age of 50, affects tooth-supporting bone.

## Poor Diet

Improper diet may influence periodontal health. Usually it takes a severe vitamin deficiency to affect a noticeable gum change. However, all the body systems and organs are influenced by the proper intake of a nutritious diet. A poor diet may alter the ability of the gum tissue to resist infection, as well as respond effectively to treatment.

# LOCAL FACTORS INFLUENCING THE PROGNOSIS

## Plaque Control

The ability to maintain low levels of plaque and the motivation to continue doing so after active treatment, are critical to success of therapy and insuring a better prognosis.

## Pocket Depth

Numerous studies have shown that the deeper the pocket the more difficult it is to treat and the more likely that there will be disease progression. Therefore, teeth with shallower pockets will generally have a better prognosis.

## Remaining Supporting Bone

The amount of remaining bone which supports the tooth is crucial. If bone loss is extensive or peculiarly shaped, the prognosis is poor.

## Number of Remaining Teeth

If the number and distribution of remaining teeth are inadequate to support replacements, such as bridges or removable partials, the prognosis is likely to be poor. The weakened teeth will be compromised by having to standing alone and absorb excess biting pressures.

## Loose teeth

Teeth that are loose due to bone loss are more likely to suffer further bone loss and develop increased sensitivity.

## Tooth Root Dimension

A long root has a greater amount of supporting bone. The loss of, let's say 1/4 inch of bone on a long root would not be as harmful as the same amount of bone loss around a short root. Molar teeth have more than one root (Fig. 6-4). *Furcation involvement,* an infection which invades the bone between the roots, creates special problems for treatment and a definite poorer prognosis.

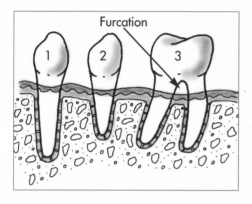

**Fig. 6-4**
Even though the level of bone loss is the same for each of these teeth, the best prognosis is for tooth "1" which has a normal well-formed root, rather than for "2" which has a short root and "3" which has a furcation involvement.

## Bad Bite

*Malocclusion* is when the teeth do not meet properly when you bite. Some absorb greater stress than they were designed for, and shift or loosen within the socket. The longer this continues, the more the teeth become weaker and sensitive. Crowded, rotated and loose teeth are also susceptible targets for plaque build-up leading to gum disease.

## Tooth Grinding

Clenching or grinding one's teeth is called *bruxism.* Many people do this unknowingly in their sleep. During bruxism, excessive pressures are generated by the facial musculature on the teeth. If this process occurs with teeth already suffering from periodontal disease, the bone loss can be accelerated.

## Poor Dental Restorations (Fillings, Crowns and Dentures)

Weakened, cracked or ill-fitting fillings and crowns lead to the accumulation of plaque, which promotes gum disease. Loose partial dentures with unstable connections to the teeth, can weaken the supporting teeth and irritate gum tissues.

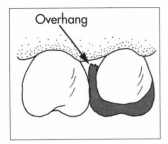

**Fig. 6-5**
OVERHANG
In this illustration, an *overhang*, a poorly shaped filling or restoration is demonstrated, which can contribute to plaque accumulation and gum disease.

## Influence of the Therapist

In addition to the local and general factors, an important influence in the overall response to treatment must include the therapist's skill and experience. Needless to say, as the disease progresses or becomes more complicated, advanced treatment is required. The therapist whose skill and experience includes the full range of periodontal treatments and diagnoses will enhance the prognosis.

## RANGE OF PROGNOSIS

An analysis is made of all the accumulated information, including the local and general influencing factors. A prediction is then made of the future of your teeth. The range of prognosis may include the following terms: Good, Fair, Guarded and Hopeless.

- **GOOD** indicates that there is strong reason to believe that the teeth will respond to periodontal therapy and may not even need advanced treatment in order to be maintained for life.

- **FAIR** indicates that the chances of success are realistic. Some bone loss has occurred; surgical therapy may be required. However, with appropriate follow-up treatment the teeth could be expected to last for many years.

- **GUARDED** (also "poor" or "questionable") would signify that even if treatment is rendered, the chances for complete success are limited. Teeth that are saved may need to be joined together for mutual support (see splinting page 92).

- **HOPELESS** means there is no reasonable possibility of being able to save the tooth; the disease is too advanced, and the damage too severe.

The most detailed prognosis includes a scenario for each tooth as well as all the teeth as one functioning unit. The prognosis clearly spells out the course the disease is likely to take, as well as the chances for the successful treatment and maintenance of the teeth. One should keep in mind that during and after treatment, the prognosis can change (for better or worse) as a result of the patient's response to therapy.

With the prognosis completed, the patient is able to begin the treatment phase.

# PART III

## *Treatment*

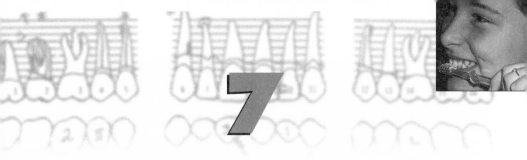

# PLAQUE CONTROL

## Everyday Care
## for Your Teeth and Gums

This is the most important topic of the book, because it deals with what you can do to help arrest your disease and save your teeth. Please read it carefully.

### The First Step

Recalling that the chief cause of gum disease is plaque, it is logical that treatment is directed towards eliminating this cause.

Unless there is an emergency, the first step in the treatment of gum disease is adopting an effective oral disease control program aimed at achieving as plaque-free a mouth as possible. Every dental professional will approach this challenge in a different way, including the use of demonstration videos and booklets to help patients understand their disease.

### What You Need to Know to Control Plaque Every Day

The single most important treatment anyone can do for gum disease is daily plaque removal performed using scientifically proven techniques.

You will probably need to change the way you clean your teeth. Old habits will have to be abandoned. New methods will be a bother, a time-consuming nuisance, until you establish new patterns. But nothing else will solve your problem. No pill has yet been produced which rids plaque from your mouth!

Look at it this way: if your present cleaning ritual was doing the job, you would have no need for periodontal treatment; you would probably not even be reading this book. So, recognizing that you need to change your methods is a good start.

You cannot clean your teeth too often. Many therapists recommend cleaning after every meal. This is perhaps an idealistic goal that few can actually achieve. Experts would agree that one thorough cleaning a day is preferable to three or more cursory ones.

How do you brush your teeth now? Up and down, as many of us were once taught? Or with a horizontal scrubbing motion that is easier and more natural? Do you use a hard brush or soft? Natural bristles or nylon? Toothpaste, gel or powder? Floss or toothpicks?

As a result of scientific studies, many of the long accepted ideas about tooth brushing have been discarded. And yet there are still many variations of accepted brushing techniques. This is because each patient's teeth are different and have unique problems with plaque control. Your therapist will give you specific instructions on the best methods for cleaning your teeth.

## Disclosing Plaque

To effectively remove plaque you need to see it. For this purpose, a disclosing solution or tablet (available at most pharmacies) is used containing a dye which identifies plaque. Patients are instructed how to apply the dye. Observing your teeth at this time will reveal areas of plaque accumulation where oral hygiene procedures need to be improved.

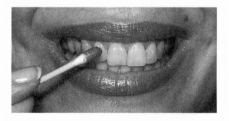

**Fig. 7-1**
Placing disclosing solution directly on the teeth will identify areas of plaque which can be easily cleaned.

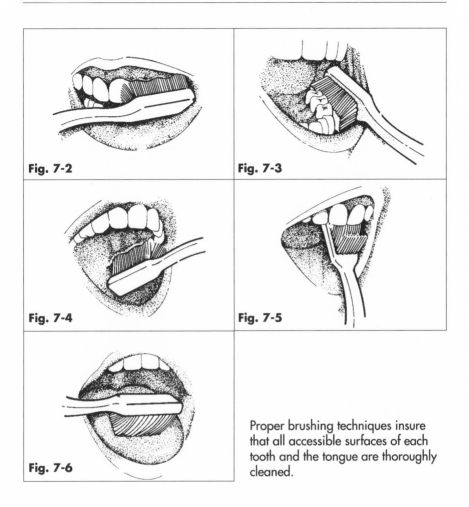

Fig. 7-2

Fig. 7-3

Fig. 7-4

Fig. 7-5

Fig. 7-6

Proper brushing techniques insure that all accessible surfaces of each tooth and the tongue are thoroughly cleaned.

## BRUSHING

First, use the toothbrush dry and with no toothpaste. Starting on the outside upper or lower molars, hold the brush parallel to the gum line and at a 45° angle to the tooth (Fig.7-2). Applying enough pressure so that the bristles can get into the sulcus between gum and tooth, brush with five or six very short strokes, just enough to move the bristles back and forth on two or three teeth at a time. It should be a vibrating motion aimed at cleaning just the area that can be covered by the bristles at one time.

After several short strokes, turn the handle of the brush in your hand so that the bristles sweep from the gum toward the top of the teeth. Then move the brush around the mouth and repeat the procedure until you have cleaned the outer side of all the teeth, top and bottom (Fig. 7-3).

Now, begin the same process on the inner side (Fig. 7-4). You will find that it is easy to jiggle the brush and sweep away from the gum on the sides. It may be more difficult to brush in the same way behind your front teeth (Fig. 7-5). For this area a smaller brush may be recommended. Don't forget to brush your tongue. Many bacteria settle within the crevices of this large muscle (Fig. 7-6). Note that toothpaste is not used during this step.

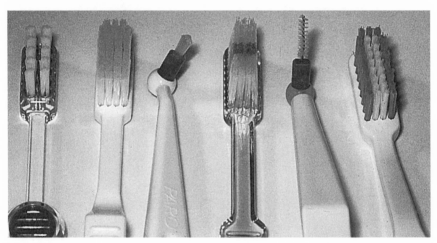

**Fig. 7-7**
Sometimes choosing from the range of toothbrush styles is overwhelming. Your therapist can recommend the right brush for you.

# FLOSSING

Most serious gum disease occurs between the teeth where brushing cannot reach. This is why so many patients who brush religiously are shocked to discover that they are in jeopardy of losing their teeth. If the space between the teeth is not cleaned, gum disease may occur. Floss is our chief weapon for this area. Many people use dental floss only to dislodge bits of food trapped between their teeth. To prevent gum disease however, flossing should be done as often as brushing or at least once a day.

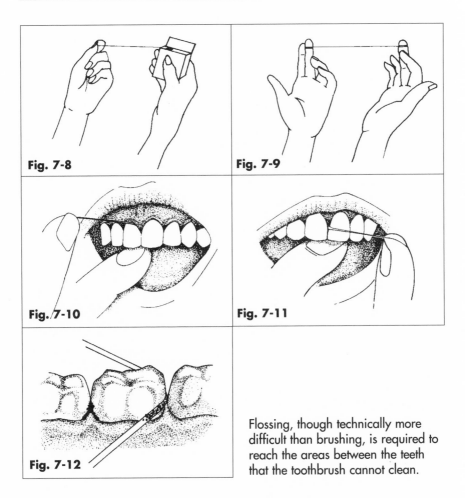

Fig. 7-8

Fig. 7-9

Fig. 7-10

Fig. 7-11

Fig. 7-12

Flossing, though technically more difficult than brushing, is required to reach the areas between the teeth that the toothbrush cannot clean.

If you do it correctly, you will use two to three feet of dental floss each time. If that seems like a lot, consider that it is just one or two inches of floss per tooth. The best approach is to hold the dental floss dispenser in one hand. Pull out about eighteen inches of floss (Fig. 7-8) and take one turn around the middle finger on the hand holding the dispenser. Now anchor the end of the floss by taking two or three turns around the middle finger of the other hand, leaving five or six inches of floss between the two hands (Fig. 7-9). Then, using both index fingers to guide the floss, place it around the sides of one of your front teeth. Bring the floss gently down into the sulcus between tooth and gum and pull the ends of the floss forward to form a tight

"C" around the base of the tooth, (Fig. 7-10) then lift the floss up along the side of the tooth toward the top and slide over to the adjacent tooth (Fig. 7-11). Floss that breaks or sheds may indicate the need to replace weak fillings or crowns.

As you finish one tooth, allow another short length of floss to pull out of the dispenser and take up the slack by taking another wrap around your middle finger. This technique provides a clean length of floss for each tooth and prevents carrying plaque from one pocket to another.

In slipping the floss between the teeth, be careful not to pull so hard that the floss is jerked into the gum. These tissues are tender and can be injured if the floss is handled too roughly. You will soon develop a routine for flossing both sides of each tooth in turn. It is not important where you start or finish. The main thing is to be sure that you remove the plaque as completely as possible from both sides of each tooth (Fig. 7-12).

## TOOTHPASTE

When flossing is finished, you are ready for toothpaste and a final brushing. Toothpaste is useful as a breath freshener and tooth polish, but it is relatively ineffective in removing plaque. This is why you need to do the plaque control steps first. Some toothpastes have additives that assist in retarding the accumulation of plaque and tartar: fluoride to reduce decay and other ingredients that can help control gingivitis.

Again, the recommended technique is to brush away from the gums toward the top of the tooth so that the bristles can sweep into the spaces between the gum and tooth. Most toothpastes are acceptable but your therapist may recommend a special toothpaste depending on your individual dental condition.

## SPECIAL DEVICES FOR IMPROVED PLAQUE CONTROL

Patients with fixed bridges or very tight spaces may find normal flossing impossible. In these areas, specially designed *loops* (Fig. 7-13) are used which thread the floss into the spaces between the teeth and/or under the bridge. *Floss holders* act like fingers making it

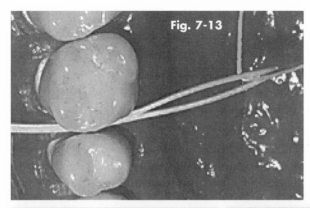

Fig. 7-13

Improving plaque control between the teeth with loops, interdental brush and woodsticks.

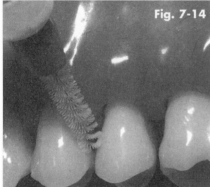

Fig. 7-14

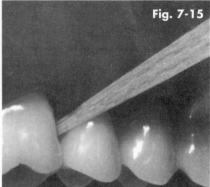

Fig. 7-15

easier to reach difficult areas with the floss. *Interdental brushes* (Fig. 7-14) are often recommended for patients as a substitute or in addition to flossing when adequate space exists between the teeth to accommodate the brush.

*Electric toothbrushes* are effective for the removal of food debris and plaque. An electric toothbrush can be helpful for the handicapped as well as for those who otherwise find it difficult to manipulate manual brushes. Some patients enjoy the novelty of the electric toothbrush, which may encourage better brushing habits. It is important to realize that regardless of the brushing technique, the plaque must be removed in order to be effective.

*Stimulating aids* such as rubber tips and woodsticks (Fig. 7-15) may be used to help firm the gum tissues through a massaging effect, and to assist in the removal of retained food particles and plaque.

## MOUTHRINSES AND ORAL IRRIGATION

Mouthrinses and other chemical solutions are often advertised as preventing bad breath. Some solutions have been shown to be effective in controlling plaque and improving gingivitis. The solutions are more efficient however, when delivered directly into the periodontal pocket by an oral irrigator. *Chlorhexidine* is one of the most widely prescribed chemical agents of this type.

Periodontists will often recommend these agents as a supplement to other therapy, when additional support for plaque control is required. The patient is instructed regarding the correct method and the period of time that these solutions are to be used. As some of the solutions are potent antimicrobial agents, it is important to follow the directions carefully, and not to undertake or change the regimen without professional consultation.

## DIET AND PERIODONTAL DISEASE

In general, a balanced diet will help to insure that your vital organs and other body systems are working at maximum efficiency. While there is little evidence of a direct correlation between general nutrition and periodontal disease, it is reasonable to assume that when a patient's general health suffers from the lack of a healthy diet, the body's ability to fight off gum infection may be impaired.

Of course, sugar specifically has a direct effect on the mouth. Not only is it responsible for dental decay but it can contribute to plaque

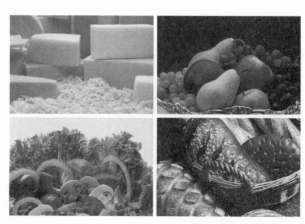

**Fig. 7-16**
A diet containing the essential food groups will contribute to overall health and may influence the health of your gums.

formation. The reader is referred to the many excellent guides to nutrition for establishing a balanced healthy diet.

## One Day At a Time

If all these changes in the care of your mouth seem like a heavy burden, perhaps it is best not to think too far in the future. Try taking one day at a time. Start with one aid and one area of the mouth and work your way up to a comprehensive routine. To check your overall brushing and flossing efficiency, try to use plaque disclosing material once every other day after oral hygiene procedures for the first two weeks, followed by once a week as a continual check.

With most periodontal diseases, you are really much more fortunate than patients suffering from the majority of medical ailments. Few can actually take direct action which will arrest or reverse their disease.

With the help of your periodontist or dentist to advise and provide treatment as necessary, the patient who develops an effective program of plaque control can cure early gum disease and better maintain the results of treatment.

# 8

# INITIAL THERAPY

## *Primary Treatment for Most Periodontal Diseases*

While the patient is learning to effectively remove plaque, a series of treatments is usually performed, aimed at reducing the causes and influences within the mouth which are responsible for periodontal disease. These procedures, which include plaque control, are non-surgical and are often collectively termed *initial therapy*.

## SCALING

In combination with plaque control, nearly all forms of gum disease are improved by removing local irritants and preventing their recurrence. The process of removing plaque and tartar from the teeth is know as *scaling*. Your dentist may have scaled your teeth as part of a procedure commonly known as *cleaning*. A cleaning however may not include scaling, especially in the case of patients without gum disease, and is often limited to a cursory removal of stain.

# ROOT PLANING

After scaling, the tooth's root is often left with a rough surface. Also there may be areas where the cementum (the outer covering of the root surface) has been softened by periodontal disease. Root planing is a delicate smoothing of the rough or irregular root's surface to enhance reattachment of gum tissues and retard plaque formation.

## For your comfort...

During scaling and root planing you may receive a local anesthetic injection or anesthetic paste to eliminate discomfort. Scaling and root planing utilize a variety of specialized instruments to remove plaque and tartar. This wide range of options makes it possible to comfortably gain access to deposits above and below the gum line. Most of the time, these procedures do not cause pain. However, some patients are nevertheless more relaxed with the area anesthetized.

Periodontists schedule from one to six or more appointments to complete scaling and root planing and may perform the treatment by segments. The segments are usually made up of quarters of the mouth known as *quadrants* (up to eight teeth). Your therapist may treat one or two quadrants at a time. Occasionally the entire mouth is completed in one session.

# POLISHING

The final smoothing of the tooth surfaces is called *polishing*. For this procedure, a polishing agent such as a paste of fine pumice is applied to a rubber polishing cup or brush. Any remaining tooth discoloration

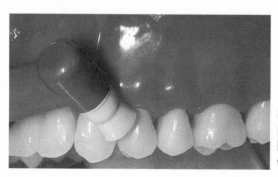

**Fig. 8-1**
Polishing removes stain and leaves a smooth surface on the teeth.

74

may be removed as well. *Fluoride* may be applied after polishing because of its ability to reduce sensitivity and its known anti-decay properties.

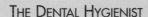

## THE DENTAL HYGIENIST

Dental hygienists are important professional members of the periodontal therapy team and may (under the direction of the periodontist) undertake partial or complete responsibility for scaling, root planing, motivation and plaque control. The dental hygienist is trained to perform a wide variety of additional duties including periodontal probing, taking of impressions for diagnostic models, x-rays and application of various medications.

## An Amazing Healing Process at Work in Your Mouth

More than anything else, successful treatment of early gum disease is predictable because of the remarkable capacity of the gum tissues to heal and repair following the removal of plaque and tartar, and improvement in oral hygiene.

Think of an embedded wood splinter that separates two sides of skin. The splinter is acting as an irritant. As long as it remains the skin will not join back together. And yet, soon after the splinter is removed, the skin begins to repair itself until the separation disappears. This is similar to what happens after scaling and root planing.

Following removal of the irritants (represented by the splinter analogy), the gum pocket fills with a microscopic blood clot and is then replaced by reparative tissue. Within a day or two, the inner gum begins to heal, and is often reattached to the tooth by the end of two weeks. Usually, if the disease is caught early enough, consistency, contour and texture of the gums will return to health, and the gum margin will adapt to the tooth.

## CORRECTING DENTAL RESTORATIONS

You may have discovered difficulty flossing in areas where old fillings or poor fitting crowns (*restorations*) were found. These problems can impede good results following scaling and root planing, and contribute to further retention of plaque. For these reasons, the correction of poor fitting restorations will, when possible, be accomplished as part of the initial procedures by your dentist in consultation with the periodontist. In addition, removal of active decay, required root canal therapy or extraction of hopeless teeth may be completed at this time.

## TREATING BITE PROBLEMS

Irregularity in the bite or malocclusion is an important consideration in the treatment of periodontal disease. When the teeth do not meet evenly or are positioned improperly in the mouth, gum disease can be exacerbated.

### Occlusal Adjustment

*Occlusal adjustment* involves the reshaping or smoothing of the tooth's biting surfaces so that the bite becomes gradually more even and the pressures balanced throughout the mouth.

For this procedure a handpiece or rotary drill is utilized that allows

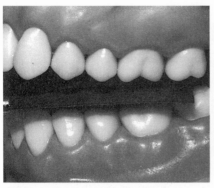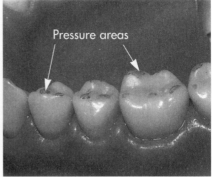

**Fig. 8-2** OCCLUSAL ADJUSTMENT
The marking paper placed between the teeth (left) identifies areas of unequal pressure (right); when these areas are "adjusted" the patient will benefit from a more comfortable bite.

a minimal amount of tooth material to be removed or reshaped.

The patient is asked to bring the teeth together during normal chewing strokes. A strip of inked, thin paper is held between the teeth. When the paper is removed, pressure points are seen where the teeth came together. The darker pressure points represent areas that need reshaping.

Occlusal adjustment is not painful. This treatment may involve one or more appointments depending on the severity of the problem. Most patients find that following occlusal adjustment their bite is more comfortable and their teeth have a sense of "belonging together."

## Bite Guard Therapy

Patients with a grinding or clenching habit called bruxism exert excessive stress on the teeth. To alleviate these problems, a bite guard is made. This removable appliance is designed from models taken of the patient's teeth. Bite guards are usually made of a hard plastic that fit over the upper or lower teeth (Fig. 8-3). The bite guard is designed to be worn during periods of bruxism. For many, this is during sleep. Others find it necessary at work or when they pursue concentrated tasks. For some, the wearing of a bite guard is required twenty-four hours a day.

Use of the bite guard may eliminate the habit of bruxism, however most patients continue to grind or clench and must wear the bite

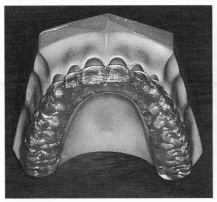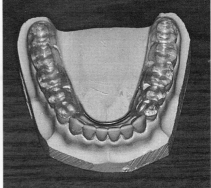

**Fig. 8-3**
A bite guard is made from a clear plastic to fit around the upper (left) or lower teeth (right).

guard for an extended period of time. Patients also often report relief from the symptoms of TM Disorders (discussed on page 46). The appliance must be checked for evidence of wear. Adjustments are often required.

## Orthodontics

*Orthodontics* (straightening of the teeth) may be included during comprehensive periodontal treatment to correct abnormalities that contribute to gum disease or for purely esthetic reasons. Adults are usually surprised to find that with modern transparent brackets and plastic wires much of the stigma associated with "braces" has been eliminated. *Minor tooth movement* is the realignment of teeth that do not require complex techniques. More involved treatment requiring the banding of all teeth, or major realignment of the teeth and jaws may be referred to an *orthodontist.*

If a patient is considering orthodontics, active gum disease must be eliminated prior to the start of treatment. The braces, brackets and wires used in orthodontics attract plaque and can result in overgrowth or infection of the gum tissue. Tooth movement in an infected area can lead to abscesses, rapid destruction of bone and the loss of teeth.

Patients with treated gum disease need to be seen frequently for periodontal monitoring during orthodontic care.

# REEVALUATION

Usually a waiting period of a few weeks to several months passes before a reevaluation is made regarding further treatment. During reevaluation, many factors are considered. If, for example, periodontal pockets have been reduced, bleeding eliminated and the patient is able to thoroughly remove plaque on a daily basis, no further treatment may be required.

On the other hand, patients with continuing problems, especially periodontal pockets greater than four millimeters, signs of inflammation and esthetic defects, will benefit from the advanced periodontal therapy discussed in the next chapter.

# 9

# ADVANCED THERAPY

## *Periodontal Surgery Options*

In advanced gum disease, surgery offers the best chance for saving teeth. Various studies have shown that the vast majority of patients who have had periodontal surgery are able to retain most if not all of their teeth. This is a reassuring statement. In some cases some very weak teeth may eventually be lost. But corrective surgery and follow-up treatment can be given credit for saving the rest. As a patient, your chances of living out your whole life with your own teeth are excellent.

### ...A Word (or two) About "The Word"

To begin with, there is clearly something about the word "surgery" that can have an unsettling effect. That is understandable. Surgery conjures up a sense of serious business. There are, of course, certain risks involved in any procedure, be it a heart transplant or a wart removal. Also, there is no getting away from the fact that any surgical procedure is unpleasant. Its aftermath almost always involves some temporary, although often surprisingly mild, discomfort. The degree of discomfort will vary with each patient.

79

Apart from the fear of pain, there are the psychological factors stimulated by the announcement that the next step is surgery. Such announcement proclaims to the patient that there is something irrevocably wrong. One can no longer think, "I'm really O.K. I just ought to remember to brush my teeth more often." The recommendation of surgery can be an attack on the patient's basic self image and triggers complex and unconscious reactions.

One may think it an indictment of the patient's ability to take proper care of one's self. It may be a grim reminder of advancing age and eventual mortality. It recalls the admonition of parents or teachers. It can awaken buried hostilities. It often suggests a measure of personal failure. All these reactions and others affect the patient's response to the need for surgery.

While most patients react with some degree of apprehension when surgery is discussed, many have found that the anticipatory fear is far outweighed by the reality of the actual experience.

Unfortunately, some people who are so paralyzed by the *sound* of the word surgery, would rather chance having false teeth than undergo the procedure. The tragedy is that these are the individuals who, because they chose not to have surgery, will likely suffer the discomfort, expense and eventual tooth loss they had hoped to avoid.

## RELAX – Reducing Stress Before and After Surgery

Despite having full confidence in their periodontist, and after all the explanations of the true nature of the advanced procedures, it is natural for some patients to still feel apprehensive prior to surgery. Reducing pre-surgery stress enables the body to relax. Allocating time away from a demanding work schedule before surgery for sports or hobbies is a good stress reducer. Remember, stress may be a contributing factor to certain types of gum disease. It may even be a significant deterrent to speedy healing. Therefore, managing your tensions may be as important as the actual operating techniques.

Though performing surgery in a very localized area, the conscientious surgeon remembers that the mouth is only a part of the total human being. Therefore, to help the patient relax prior and during surgery, the following additional suggestions may be considered.

## Medications

For patients apprehensive about surgery, tranquilizers or sedatives can be prescribed. Some are taken the night before; others are taken or injected while resting in the office prior to or during the procedure. These medications will calm your fears and allow you to be more relaxed.

## Nitrous Oxide (Laughing Gas)

One of the most popular of all the relaxing agents used in dentistry is *nitrous oxide/oxygen*. Nitrous oxide was known as laughing gas in the 1800's when first used as a form of entertainment in circuses (see page 19). However, in the dental office it is combined with oxygen and inhaled through a nose mask promoting a dreamlike sensation, euphoria, and a feeling of well-being for the anxious patient. Nitrous oxide with oxygen does not produce an unconscious state. Patients are most definitely awake but are frequently heard to say, "I know you are doing something but it really doesn't matter."

## Full Mouth Surgery and Hospital Care

The idea of "getting it all over with at once" may be appealing and can be accomplished in the specially equipped periodontal office or hospital operating room.

Patients who select this approach are given either general anesthesia or a milder sedation which promotes a sense of detachment and calm during the procedure.

The surgical techniques themselves are the same, regardless of whether performed in segments or at one time. The full mouth procedure however may last two to four hours and would involve a more uncomfortable and slightly longer recovery period than expected of the patient having segmental surgery.

## SURGERY FOR DEEP OR DIFFICULT-TO-CLEAN POCKETS

Patients with deep, difficult-to-clean pockets and/or continuing signs of inflammation (Fig. 9-1) are unable to effectively fight the accumulation of plaque and more likely to experience progression of their disease. The benefits of periodontal surgery in these cases include improved ability to perform effective plaque control, halting the continual deepening of pockets, rebuilding lost support and prevention of tooth loss.

Generally, only part of your mouth will be treated at a single sitting. If one quadrant (one quarter of the mouth) or one half of the mouth is treated, the patient can still eat comfortably and perform regular plaque control on the untreated side.

After arrival at the periodontist's office, the patient is encouraged to become as comfortable as possible in the dental chair. You can loosen your collar or belt, perhaps even remove your shoes. In addition to any relaxation options you may have chosen, a local anesthetic will be given. No pain will be felt.

The periodontist is assisted by a nurse or dental assistant who is not

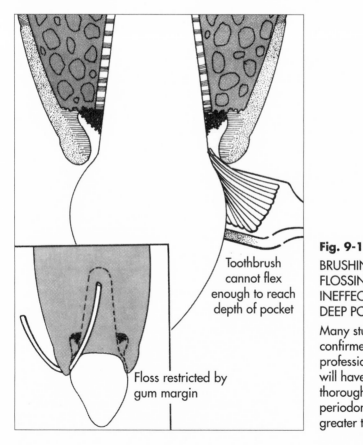

Toothbrush cannot flex enough to reach depth of pocket

Floss restricted by gum margin

**Fig. 9-1**

BRUSHING AND FLOSSING ARE INEFFECTIVE IN DEEP POCKETS

Many studies have confirmed that even a professional therapist will have difficulty to thoroughly clean periodontal pockets greater than 4mm.

82

only trained to help technically during the procedure, but also is particularly concerned about the patient's comfort.

One or a combination of several corrective procedures will be chosen to treat the deep pockets.

## GINGIVECTOMY – GINGIVOPLASTY

*Gingivectomy* is the removal of gingival or gum tissue, just as appendectomy is removal of the appendix. At one time, it was the most widely used type of periodontal surgery. This procedure reduces the depth of periodontal pockets and at the same time exposes the calculus or tartar for more effective removal. The gingivectomy may be the preferred procedure in cases of swollen gums. Gingivectomy is usually performed when there is no bone loss, and is therefore not generally employed in advanced cases. In the past, over-utilization of the gingivectomy removed much of the protective gum (gingiva) tissue. *Gingivoplasty* refers to the reshaping or sculpturing of the gum tissues. These minor adjustments will improve esthetics and/or enhance the ability to perform effective plaque control.

## FLAP PROCEDURES

Most advanced cases of gum disease will predictably benefit from a *flap procedure.* As the name implies, a delicate incision separating the periodontal pockets and gum tissue from the tooth creates a flap of gum tissue. There may be an inner flap consisting of the gum tissue on the tongue side of the tooth, or an outer flap developed from the gum on the cheek side of the tooth. Most frequently both areas are treated in this manner. What makes this procedure special? Unlike gingivectomy where gum tissue is removed, this procedure preserves the gum tissue which is returned to its place at the end of the surgery. Little or no gum tissue is lost.

The main advantage however, of this sophisticated flap approach is that it provides access to the underlying diseased structures. Once the incision has been made, several delicate steps will follow. The flaps are gently separated from the teeth and bone so that the meticulous step of the procedure can be accomplished: the removal of all the diseased tissue, calculus, and other pocket remnants located in the small convoluted defects within the bone.

Following thorough removal of all diseased tissue, the root surfaces are scaled and smoothed. The surgery may be completed at this point or continued with treatment of the underlying bone.

## TREATING PROBLEMS IN THE BONE

Periodontitis results in formation of defects between the bone and the roots of the teeth, which become a focal area for reinfection. In many cases, treatment of the underlying bone or *osseous* defects, is considered an essential part of managing periodontal disease. With the flap raised and undesirable tissues removed, the bone surrounding the defects is directly visible and treatable.

### Bone Reshaping

This procedure reduces thick margins which project from the bone around the teeth and improves the positioning of the replaced flaps. Small amounts of bone around the defects and adjacent teeth may also be removed to enhance the healing and assist in reducing pockets.

### Root Removal

Molars, which have two or three roots sometimes suffer bone loss between the roots known as furcation involvement (Fig. 6-4). When there is no alternative, removal of the root with the most bone loss may be elected to allow the healthier remaining part of the tooth to survive. A *root canal* which involves removing the tooth's nerve and other components of the dental pulp (Fig. 2-2) is performed either prior to or directly after this procedure. Afterwards, a crown is often recommended.

### Regeneration: For New Tooth-Supporting Tissues

One of the more advanced methods for treating bone defects is known as *regeneration;* the growth of cells to form new tissues which replace missing or damaged ones. This process goes on naturally throughout our bodies providing replacement tissues for those that become old and die. As we age, this process becomes slower and less efficient. But usually it is still working well enough throughout our lifetime to repair our cuts and bruises.

In the past, predictable regeneration of tooth-supporting tissues (bone, root cementum, and attaching fibers) was only a dream. The periodontal defect being under constant attack by bacterial plaque, food debris and retained calculus was a difficult area to expect good results.

Today, however, use of the advanced procedures discussed in this next section have turned regeneration into a reality.

## Bone Replacement Grafting

Various materials can be placed into the bone defect in a fashion similar to puttying up a hole in your wall. The bone replacement graft becomes incorporated into the defect and/or replaced by the patient's own bone during healing. Bone grafting material can be acquired from a number of different sources.

- ### The Patient's Bone

  The patient's own bone is an excellent and convenient grafting material. Bits of bone shavings collected during periodontal surgery can be placed directly into the bone defects. A recent extraction space or other areas of the mouth can also be excellent sources of graft material.

- ### Donated Origin

  Freeze-dried donor bone can be procured from tissue banks, which also supply bone for many routine medical procedures. Qualified tissue banks insure that donated bone undergoes vigorous screening, testing and special techniques to eradicate the possibility of disease or infection transmission. This bone can be used alone or mixed with the patient's own bone, as a combined grafting material.

- ### Bone Substitutes

  Synthetic or organic-derived materials may also be placed into the bone defect. These substances can act in a manner similar to human bone grafts, as a filler to maintain space for regeneration, or serve principally to stimulate the growth of new bone and attachment.

## Membranes-Guided Tissue Regeneration (GTR)

Regeneration techniques often incorporate a *membrane* either alone or in combination with bone grafting, in a process called *guided tissue regeneration* or GTR, see below. GTR means that the type of tissue we want to grow (in this case, bone and fiber attachments) is guided by the exclusion of the tissue we don't want (gum and other soft tissues).

By covering the defect, the membrane can promote GTR as well as contain the graft within the defect. Membranes are made of various materials. Some are self-dissolving, while others require a second surgical procedure to be removed.

**Fig. 9-2**

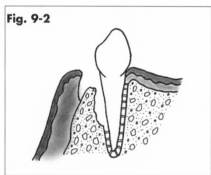

**Fig. 9-3**

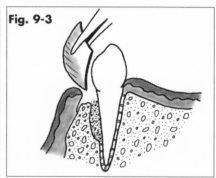

**Fig. 9-4**

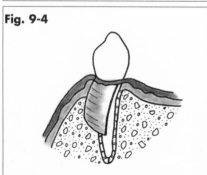

**Fig. 9-5**

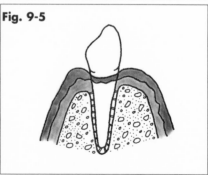

COMBINATION REGENERATION PROCEDURES

In this series, the bone defect and root surfaces have been thoroughly cleaned (Fig. 9-2). A bone substitute or graft material is placed, while a self-dissolving membrane is prepared (Fig. 9-3), and then draped over the area (Fig. 9-4). Within three months, new bone and possible attachments (Fig. 9-5) can be expected to replace a substantial part of the previous defect.

### Influencing Successful Regeneration

The overall success of regeneration techniques has been very promising. The factors which influence the success of these procedures include the materials used, the type of defects treated, the control of risk factors, such as smoking and the surgeon's ability and experience.

# COSMETIC PERIODONTAL SURGERY
## Making Your Smile Healthy *and* Beautiful

The mouth is the most expressive part of you face. Sadness, fear, exultation and allure are all remarkably communicated to someone via the mouth.

Few things are more pleasing to the eye than a beautiful smile. A beautiful smile radiates health, vitality, warmth and yes, sex appeal. Cosmetic periodontal surgery procedures correct problems in the relationship between the teeth, gum and surrounding tissues that often are the cause of an unattractive smile.

## CROWN LENGTHENING: Correcting "Short" Teeth

An individual may appear to have short teeth only to discover that the teeth are of normal length but burdened with an abundance of gum tissue, sometimes referred to as a "gummy smile." These patients have suffered for years, hiding their teeth due to embarrassment either because they thought their teeth were too small or showed too much

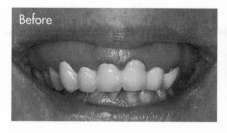 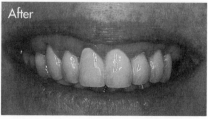

**Fig. 9-6** CROWN LENGTHENING
This patient was reluctant to smile due to the exposure of excess gum tissues (left). Two weeks after crown lengthening and the placement of temporary crowns, there is a dramatic improvement.

gum while smiling. The benefits of cosmetic surgery (gingivectomy or a flap procedure) are immediate and dramatic as the full natural, attractive smile is revealed.

Crown lengthening increases tooth length. The word "crown" refers to that part of the tooth normally present above the gum line. Although crown lengthening is always required to increase the length of the tooth for esthetics, it may also be prescribed by your dentist when the available tooth structure is too short to prepare for caps or crowns.

## GUM REPLACEMENT GRAFTS
### For Weak Gums and Exposed Roots

Gum recession and its associated root exposure can be very unpleasant especially when it appears in the front of the mouth. Exposed roots can also make an individual look older than his real age, as well as lead to sensitivity and cavities. In addition, when the quality of the gum is poor, these fragile tissues can become easily inflamed or damaged from injury leading to root exposure.

Techniques for grafting gum or compatible soft tissues within the mouth have made it possible to reinforce areas of weak gum tissues and frequently cover exposed roots. Gum grafts may also be indicated to strengthen gum tissues associated with planed crowns, bridges and orthodontic treatment.

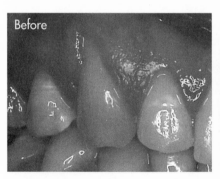
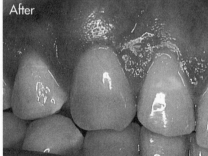

**Fig. 9-7** COVERING EXPOSED ROOT
This twenty-one year old was always self-conscious about her recession and root exposure. After a successful gum graft, the root is covered and the new tissue blends perfectly with the adjacent gums.

## Types of Gum Grafts

There are two major types of gum grafts: *pedicle* grafts remain partially attached to the donor site and are therefore limited to close proximity defects. *Free* grafts are completely detached from their source and can be utilized anywhere in the mouth. Free grafts are usually taken from the palate. Sometimes the two procedures are combined.

## Repairing Gum Indentations

Unsightly indentations in the gums may occur after tooth removal or as a result of accident or diseases. These defects themselves are not only disfiguring but cause the replacement tooth to be out of proportion and unattractive in comparison with the remaining teeth. Special techniques are utilized to repair and fill in these types of esthetic defects by combining gum and sometimes bone grafting procedures.

## FRENECTOMY

The *frenum* is composed of muscle-like fibers extending from the lip and cheek to the gums (Fig. 9-8). Frenum can contribute to recession of the gum margin, root exposure and pain during normal brushing. A frenum attached too closely to the gum margin can open the walls of an existing periodontal pocket during talking and eating, and retard good healing following surgery. In these situations, removal of

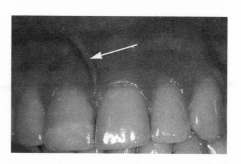

**Fig. 9-8**
THE FRENUM
Though located in several areas of mouth, a frenum is most often noticed connecting to the gum tissues just above the two upper central teeth.

the frenum or *frenectomy* is recommended. There is no harm in being without a frenum. A frenectomy is frequently incorporated with other surgical techniques or during orthodontic treatment to aid in the movement of teeth and enhance their stability.

## Smile Consultation

It may be surprising to discover just how many esthetics problems in the mouth can be resolved after consulting with a periodontist. Looking at your smile together, you and the periodontist can review the specific procedures that will enable you to achieve the smile you always wanted.

# CONCLUDING PROCEDURES AND FOLLOW UP CARE

The following procedures are generally performed at the conclusion of surgery.

## Replacement of Flaps and Suturing

The replaced flaps or grafted tissues are *sutured* (sewed) to maintain the flaps in position. Some sutures are removed during a postoperative visit while others, made of biodegradable material are self-dissolving.

## Periodontal Dressing

A periodontal dressing may be used. This surgical dressing is a mixture of materials that have the initial consistency of putty. It is easily shaped around the surgery area and between the teeth. Afterwards, the dressing becomes firm and will be removed at a later visit.

## Post-operative Instructions

Post-operative instructions contain important information about how to care for your mouth after surgery, such as where and how to brush, recommended foods to eat and the telephone number to call with any questions. You will receive a prescription for the relief of any discomfort, as well as antibiotics and a medicated mouth rinse if appropriate for the procedure.

Patients usually return in a week to ten days for their first post-operative visit, which includes examination, removal of any periodontal dressing and sutures (if they are not self-dissolving), special oral hygiene instructions and other procedures that may assist the healing process.

## Discomfort

For the record, let us face the question of discomfort head on. Yes, the surgical procedure may be unpleasant, but it is not painful. Today, besides the possible annoyance of the anesthetic needle, the only real discomfort is having to hold your mouth open long enough and sometimes wide enough to complete the treatment.

After the anesthetic wears off, you may experience somewhat of a sore mouth and possibly minor swelling. However, with medication, the discomfort is considerably minimized. Many patients are back to normal activities the following day. Soreness can occasionally last a bit longer for some, depending on the exact nature and extent of the surgery.

## Changes in the Mouth After Periodontal Surgery

With successful periodontal surgery, many welcome changes occur in the gum tissues, including reduced pockets and elimination of active inflammation, as well as a clean, fresh feeling in the mouth. Other changes, generally as a result of flap or gingivectomy surgery, may be of concern to the patient at first and are described below.

- **Movement of the Gum Line.** Sometimes the gum line heals farther away from its position prior to surgery. This is the result of eliminating diseased materials that created an infected layer between the gum and the bone. After surgery, the healthy gum lays above the bone without any imposed infected tissue. In the front of the mouth, surgical procedures can be modified to avoid or reduce the shift of the gum line.

- **Food Catches.** As a result of the change in the gum line, food previously collected within the gum pockets will now be found between the top of the gum and the tooth itself. Patients often refer to this area as "spaces between the teeth." The food is now exposed and easily accessible for cleaning... a far better situation than existed previously when trapped food particles quietly contributed to gum disease.

- **Tooth Sensitivity.** During the first weeks after periodontal surgery, patients may notice sensitivity to certain foods and temperature extremes along the teeth. Generally this sensitivity will diminish over time. If sensitivity continues it can be remedied by application of a medication to the area.

- **Loose Teeth.** Immediately following surgery, the teeth may seem more loose than previously. This is normal. The teeth will tighten to at least the same degree of firmness as before surgery, and often firmer. If teeth are still loose after treatment because of extensive bone loss or trauma, *splinting* techniques are used to join weak teeth to adjacent firmer teeth making one strong combined unit. Splinting methods vary from the use of reinforced glue or bonding, to crowning the teeth to be splinted.

## All things considered...

The majority of patients see these inconveniences as minor annoyances along the road to saving their teeth. Especially when one considers that a patient who refuses surgery may experience recurrent abscesses, sore gums, loose teeth, expensive dental treatment to support failing teeth, and ultimately the loss of their teeth.

## Success of Periodontal Surgery

The long term success rate in periodontal surgery is excellent, with studies over many years showing that patients who completed this treatment have kept most, if not all of their teeth. The earlier in the stage of periodontal disease that surgery can begin, the less surgery is required.

It is definitely to the patient's advantage to seek help early. Indeed, even when periodontitis is advanced, surgery offers a very real hope for the continued longevity and enjoyment of your natural teeth.

## Who Should Not Have Periodontal Surgery?

Occasionally, patients with significant periodontal disease may not be good surgery candidates for the following reasons:

- **Unwillingness to Commit to Oral Hygiene Program**
  Patients who are unwilling to develop a basic regimen of preventive oral hygiene are not candidates for surgery. Even after successful treatment, there is no immunity from gum disease. It can return without good plaque control and regular visits to the periodontist.

- **Medical Complications**

  Medical problems such as unstable diabetes, AIDS, or bleeding disorders may contraindicate surgery. Patients who are pregnant, undergoing extreme stress, are severely debilitated, psychologically impaired or who have had a recent heart attack, require special consideration prior to surgery. Surgery is not performed on patients who are uncontrolled alcoholics or drug abusers.

- **Patient Medications**

  Certain medications may cause an altered reaction to surgery and may need to be adjusted with the physician's cooperation in order to proceed with surgery. These medications include blood thinners, antidepressants, thyroid replacements, steroids and various cancer drugs.

- **Teeth with Hopeless Prognosis**

  If deterioration has progressed so far that even the most advanced procedures cannot repair the devastating results of periodontal disease, a hopeless situation exists. The tooth or teeth should be removed.

## ALTERNATIVES TO SURGERY IN ADVANCED DISEASE

In advanced periodontal disease, modern surgery is the most efficient and predictable means of reducing pocket depths, eliminating periodontal disease and ultimately keeping your natural teeth.

The following alternatives however, may be presented to you for consideration.

### Scaling, Root Planing and Oral Hygiene Only

These initial therapy procedures may be suggested as an alternative to periodontal surgery, and are sometimes referred to as *soft tissue management*. The support for this approach is based on research conducted in university settings where there was strict control on patient acceptance and unlimited time for treatment. Their results, when followed by professional check-ups every three to six months, while positive, have been difficult to replicate in private practice.

## Very Frequent Professional Care

It has been suggested by a number of studies that the need for surgery could be overcome with frequent professional care which includes initial scaling and root planing, but most importantly repetitive oral hygiene and reinforcement procedures as often as every two weeks. Theoretically, this method can work if a relatively plaque-free mouth is maintained. From a practical point of view however, the required frequency of visits is often too demanding for patients to maintain.

## Medications

Various medications and solutions have been recommended to resolve gum problems including antibiotics, anti-inflammatory agents, antiseptics, mixtures of baking soda, salt and peroxide, mouthwashes and saltwater rinses. Some medications are taken systemically while others are placed directly into the pockets by irrigating appliances or via special time-releasing carriers such as gels and strings. Some toothpastes contain ingredients that can reduce gingivitis. While certain solutions or drugs, especially antibiotics, are recommended to supplement the treatment of gum disease, to date there is no significant support for any of these materials as a stand-alone, replacement therapy.

### WHAT ARE THE LIMITATIONS TO THE SURGICAL ALTERNATIVES?

The major limitation to the success of the "Alternatives to Surgery" is the fact that reaching and thoroughly treating deep pockets with scaling, root planing and/or medications is extremely difficult, even in the hands of the most skilful professionals. There is simply a problem of physical access to these plaque infected areas (Fig. 9-1), often compounded by the anatomical barriers created by the tooth itself. Most studies have shown that deeper pockets are more likely to deteriorate. In addition, when initial improvement was noted with these methods, the occurrences of relapse have been more frequent than with surgical care.

## The Combination Approach

When surgery has been contraindicated or needs to be postponed, a combination of the above alternatives is likely to be the most effective treatment prescribed by your periodontist for deep, difficult-to-clean periodontal pockets and unresolved signs of inflammation. In this case, the fundamental goal for therapy may not be to eliminate the disease, but rather to contain it for as long as possible.

## Too Many Options?

Sometimes the many treatment options can be confusing. You should speak candidly with your periodontist. He or she is the specialist uniquely qualified to discuss with you the advantages and disadvantages of each of the various therapies.

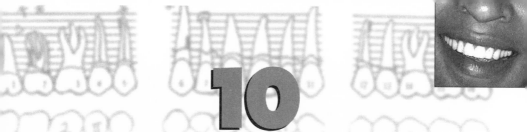

# 10

# DENTAL IMPLANTS

## Modern Solutions for Toothless Spaces

G enerally, missing teeth (other than wisdom teeth) should be replaced in order to balance the biting pressures, retain chewing efficiency and maintain the position of the remaining teeth in your mouth. The replacements will stabilize the mouth by keeping contact between teeth and reducing the possibility of shifting and rotation. At one time, replacements necessitated damage to healthy remaining teeth for support. If the patient was totally toothless, he or she would suffer the potential embarrassment of ill-fitting dentures.

Now, there is an alternative to the age-old solutions of toothless spaces: predictable *dental implants*. Just as with other body parts, teeth can be replaced with implant-supported *prostheses* (substitute artificial teeth). The result is a natural-looking improvement in your ability to talk, eat and smile with confidence.

### Types of Dental Implants

Dental implants are usually made of the same biocompatible, titanium metal used in many other types of implants throughout the body. The dental implant replaces the tooth root, and is connected to different prostheses that serve as substitutes for missing teeth. The two major categories of implants are *endosseous*, that are placed within the jaw bone, and *subperiosteal* that are placed on the bone just below the gum.

## IMPLANTS ARE VERY MUCH LIKE TEETH

Most implants in use today are endosseous or placed in the bone (about 1/2 to 3/4 inch). Because they are similar in appearance and size to the tooth root being replaced, this type of implant is also referred to as a *root form implant*. The implant may be threaded like a screw or cylinder shaped (Fig. 10-1B) and contain small vents or holes. The texture of the dental implant's outer surface can be smooth, machine roughened, coated or any combination thereof. Your periodontist can discuss with you the benefits of the various designs.

Once the implant becomes firmly attached to the surrounding bone (technically this is called *osseointegration*), an extension-base is added to the implant *(abutment)* on which the artificial tooth or prosthesis is placed.

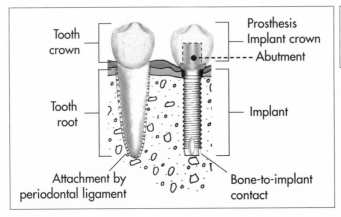

**Fig. 10-1B**
These implants, shown at *actual size*, are the most popular root form types: threaded (left) and cylinder (right).

**Fig. 10-1A**
A root form implant replaces the tooth's root; the root's size and shape are similar to the implant. The part of the tooth seen above the gum line is called the crown. The "crown" of the implant is an artificial tooth or prosthesis made of two separate units; the abutment is directly connected to the implant and the unit that appears as a tooth, fits over the abutment.

# IMPLANT ALTERNATIVES TO TRADITIONAL TOOTH REPLACEMENTS

## Instead of Altering Healthy Teeth to Make a Fixed Bridge

A *fixed bridge* is a traditional method for replacing missing teeth especially in small spaces where natural teeth are present on either side. The bridge is formed by connecting crowns (caps), that slip over altered teeth on either side of the toothless space, to a middle false tooth or teeth. The main disadvantage of the traditional bridge is that healthy natural teeth have to be shaved down to fit the connecting crowns.

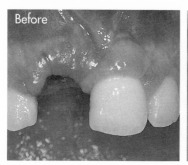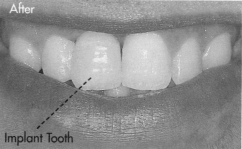

**Fig. 10-2**
MISSING TEETH REPLACED WITHOUT DAMAGING HEALTHY ONES
Replacing this patient's missing front tooth (left) with a fixed bridge would have required shaving down healthy teeth on either side. The implant solution is not only esthetic and comfortable, but preserves the natural quality of the adjacent teeth. If the patient had additional missing teeth or wanted to replace a removable partial denture, several implants would be placed, covered by individual crowns or connected as an implant-supported bridge.

Instead of altering healthy teeth to accommodate a bridge, a single dental implant is placed in the toothless space. If more than one tooth is missing several implants can be placed. The artificial teeth are then securely fitted to the implants with either tiny screws or cement; they cannot be removed by the patient. The implant alternative has many advantages including the look and feel of natural teeth, preserving the health of the remaining teeth and more efficient plaque control.

99

## In Place of Removable Partial Dentures

Removable *partial* dentures are constructed on a metal frame, covered by a gum-simulating plastic which holds the artificial teeth. This type of prosthesis is supported by a combination of the toothless ridge and the remaining teeth via metal clasps or other attachments. Patients may report that partial dentures are like having a "mouthful of hardware," are difficult to wear and feel unnatural. Sometimes, pressure from the partial denture attachments can weaken the natural teeth.

As an alternative, a fixed or permanent-type prosthesis can be made with implants placed in the position of the missing teeth. In effect, this solution is an expanded version of the individual implant technique described previously (Fig.10-2). When more than one tooth is missing, implants can be utilized to anchor an implant-supported bridge.

## To Add Support and Stability to Removable Full Dentures

A removable *full* denture replaces all the natural teeth and therefore is completely dependent on the toothless jaw for support and stability. While some patients have successfully worn removable full dentures, many complain about feeling self-conscious due to denture wobbling, clicking and pain, as well as loss of taste and poor eating ability. An implant-denture can help in one of two ways:

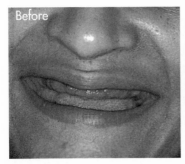
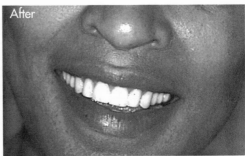

**Fig. 10-3**
THE NATURAL-LOOKING SOLUTION TO TOTAL TOOTH LOSS
This patient was embarrassed, having suffered the loss of all her teeth (left), but with an implant-supported denture, she can restore the appearance and comfort of her natural smile.

- With an adequate number of implants (up to six to eight per jaw), a *fixed-implant* denture, secured by screws or cement to the implants will restore the feeling and function similar to the natural set of teeth. This prosthesis cannot be removed by the patient. A dental professional however, may periodically remove the prosthesis for examination.

- If a fixed solution is not possible, an *implant-retained* denture will dramatically increase the stability and confidence in wearing a traditional full denture. The implants, acting as anchors, are connected to the denture by hidden attachments. This type of prosthesis is removed by the patient for inspection and cleaning.

# THE DENTAL IMPLANT PROCEDURE

## The Dental Implant Team

An excellent approach to the placement of dental implants and the final prosthesis (artificial teeth) is the *Implant Team,* that allows patients to benefit from the special expertise of each team member. The implant team works closely to coordinate the various aspects of the implant therapy.

The patient is usually unaware of the extensive consultations that often transpire between team members prior to and after the actual implant procedure. The results however, of this professional cooperation, will help to insure the correct treatment plan for each individual and contribute to the overall success of the implant.

A periodontist, the recognized expert in the gum and bone tissues that surround and support the implant, routinely performs a wide variety of sophisticated surgical procedures. This combination of knowledge and skill makes the periodontal specialist the ideal member of the team to place your implants.

The prosthetic aspect is completed by a dentist experienced in implant prostheses. This will likely be your general dentist. If he or she does not perform implant prostheses or if your mouth is particularly complicated, you will be referred to someone with the necessary skill and understanding.

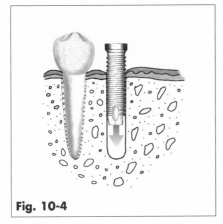

**Fig. 10-4**

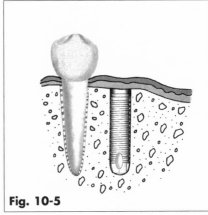

**Fig. 10-5**

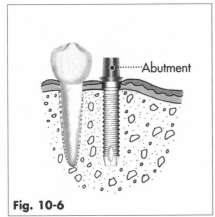

Abutment

**Fig. 10-6**

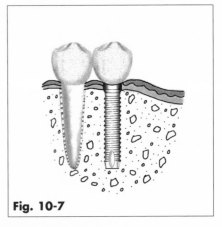

**Fig. 10-7**

## FROM IMPLANT PLACEMENT TO COMPLETED PROSTHESIS

The implant is inserted into a precisely prepared space which meets the exact dimensions of the implant (Fig. 10-4). The completely seated implant will remain undisturbed slightly above or below the gum line, until firm attachment is achieved (Fig. 10-5). After three to six months the top of the implant is uncovered and an abutment is placed (Fig. 10-6). Finally the prosthetic tooth portion is attached (Fig. 10-7).

## Getting Started

The preparatory steps prior to implant placement are similar to periodontal surgery including a thorough medical and dental history, oral exam, x-rays and possibly plaster molds of your teeth. The molds may be used by your dentist to create a surgical template which guides the periodontist when placing the implants. The use of more detailed radiographs such as CT x-ray, may be recommended to enhance the evaluation of the surgical site. A consultation with all members of the implant team will take place to coordinate each stage of the treatment.

## First Stage: Implant Placement

The anesthesia and relaxation techniques are similar to periodontal surgery. In this case, a flap (see page 83) is made and the implant receptor site fashioned in the bone to precisely accommodate the implant's dimensions. The implant is then either gently pushed or rotated into the prepared site (Fig. 10-4).

The surgery will be completed with suturing and a review of post-operative instructions, not unlike periodontal surgery. After the implant surgery however, patients with removable dentures may have to leave them out of their mouths for a short period. Additional dietary limitations may be prescribed. Return visits will be scheduled for check-ups and, if required, suture removal. The implants remain undisturbed either below or just above the gum tissues to promote the firm attachment (osseointegration) needed between implant and bone (Fig. 10-5). A temporary bridge or denture may be worn during this period in place of the missing teeth.

## Second Stage: Preparation for Prosthesis

After approximately three to six months, if the top of the implant is not protruding through the gum, a small opening is made by the periodontist to reveal the top of the implant. This is a relatively short procedure performed with local anesthesia. A protective cover or an immediate abutment is then placed on the implant.

## Third Stage: Placement of the Prosthesis

The dentist will remove the protective cover (if placed) to access the inner implant area and permit attachment of those parts that will form the prosthesis or artificial tooth. These parts include the abutment (Fig. 10-6) that attaches directly to the implant and the prosthetic crown (artificial tooth) or denture. All implant parts are made to fit the exact size and shape implant your periodontist placed during the first stage. The final texture, size, color and shape of the replacement prosthesis (Fig. 10-7) will be designed to blend with any remaining natural teeth and your general facial features.

## AUGMENTATION – For Improved Implant Placement

Previously, a lack of adequate quality or quantity of bone meant a patient could not have implants placed. Today, however augmentation procedures can enhance areas of deficient bone and improve positioning of the implant. These procedures usually require bone grafting and membrane placement (see page 86). The rate of success is good. However, the waiting period before the prosthesis can be attached may be extended from six to twelve months.

Situations that may benefit from the use of these special procedures include the following:

- ### Thin or Defective Jaw Bones

  Jaws that are too thin, deformed or have been damaged as a result of an accident or disease, can be repaired and enlarged.

- ### During Tooth Removal

  Hopeless teeth may be removed and an implant placed immediately. Sometimes, only augmentation is possible at the time of tooth removal to prepare the area for a future implant.

- ### Sinus Proximity

  The *sinus* is an air passage that rests within the bone area at about the level of your cheek just below the eye socket. A common limitation to implant therapy in the back of the upper jaw is a low sinus i.e. the sinus is too close to the implant area. To solve this problem, the lower part of the sinus is raised and the air space replaced with grafted material (*sinus lift*) allowing implants to be placed at a later stage.

## Risks

The possibility that an implant will not "take" is small, but it nevertheless exists. If an implant however should not be successful, a replacement implant can often be inserted. Other rare problems, such as temporary or extended loss of sensation or infection can occur when usually distant nerves or other anatomical areas are involved. In the event that your periodontist anticipates an area of special concern, a full explanation of these matters will be added to the discussion of the risks and benefits that precedes the placement of any dental implant.

## When Dental Implants May Not Be Recommended

Other than not having the adequate quality and quantity of bone, there are additional considerations that could limit or contraindicate recommending dental implants.

- **Medical Condition.** Any medical condition or medications, that might influence the patient's ability to have periodontal surgery will be of equal concern to the implant patient and the peri-odontist.

- **Smoking.** Smoking can jeopardize the success of implants. The patient's willingness to stop or reduce smoking should be addressed prior to the decision to have implants.

- **Gum Disease.** Implants are not placed in a mouth with untreated, active gum disease. The gum infection can contribute to the fail-ure of the most skillfully placed implants. With certain excep-tions, such as in conjunction with tooth removal, periodontal dis-ease must be under control prior to implant therapy.

- **Poor Oral Hygiene.** Oral hygiene must be adequate to assure that the gums around the implants stay healthy. The remaining natur-al teeth must also be kept as free as possible from plaque build-up and food debris.

## Dental Implant Success

Studies confirm that tested and approved implant systems used by well-trained specialists yield high rates of success. No longer must patients suffer the discomfort and humiliation of unstable and awk-ward traditional tooth replacements. Instead, they can start enjoying the many benefits of modern dental implants including a natural, secure smile with confident, comfortable eating and speech.

## IF THE FIRST U.S. PRESIDENT COULD HAVE HAD DENTAL IMPLANTS

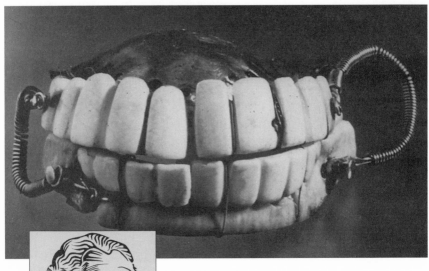

**Fig. 10-8**
While George Washington is remembered for many great attributes, his smile is not one of them. Probably, the reason was these uncomfortable spring-controlled ivory and metal dentures he had to wear. An implant prosthesis would have probably improved his disposition and his smile.

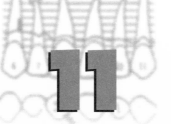

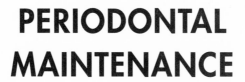

# PERIODONTAL MAINTENANCE

## Keeping Your Smile Healthy

The potential for infection and pocket formation in the treated patient is as great as before the patient had periodontal disease. There is one important difference: the periodontal patient has already demonstrated a susceptibility to gum disease and therefore may have a repeat problem. A vigorous monitored program to insure a clean mouth with minimal plaque is essential. For patients who have had implants the concern is the same, as bacteria and conditions that cause gum disease could mean serious problems for the implants as well.

### DETERMINING THE MAINTENANCE SCHEDULE

Periodontists provide a program of reevaluation and treatment visits termed *Supportive Periodontal Therapy, Periodontal Maintenance* or just *Maintenance*. Maintenance treatments begin soon after completion of active therapy and are carefully planned to accommodate the unique needs of each patient.

Studies have demonstrated that a minimum of two to three months between maintenance visits will generally significantly reduce the chances of the return of gum disease. During the first year, however, following active treatment, the patient's plaque control ability will often fluctuate while establishing acceptable intervals between maintenance visits. This is because patients require time to establish a safe period during which plaque can be adequately controlled. During this period, a patient's visits may be as frequent as bi-weekly or monthly. The frequency will be influenced by:

- the severity of the periodontal disease
- the type of treatment that was rendered
- the number of implants placed and type of prosthesis
- the results of treatment
- the effectiveness of the patient's personal plaque control
- the extent of restorative treatments (bridges, crowns etc.).

Sometimes, when the gum disease is mild, the periodontist and general dentist alternate maintenance visits.

Most specialists employ certified dental hygienists (Fig. 11-1) who play a major role in providing maintenance care, under the periodontist's supervision and guidance. Dental hygienists have enhanced experience and knowledge in the special requirements of periodontal patients.

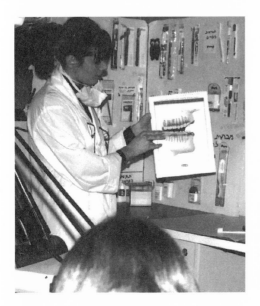

**Fig. 11-1**
The dental hygienist will often take a major role in the maintenance care of periodontal patients. One of the most significant and challenging tasks will be consistent reinforcement of effective plaque control.

# PERIODONTAL MAINTENANCE TREATMENTS

Periodontal maintenance treatments will include many of the following services during each visit:

- Review all aspects of the completed treatment
- Monitor areas with special problems
- Update medical status and medication regimen
- Check for bleeding and mobility
- Probe periodontal pockets and compare with earlier measurements
- Test to identify areas of suspected bacterial involvement
- Review flossing, brushing, and the use of plaque control aids
- Remove plaque and tartar – scaling
- Smooth root surfaces – root planing
- Polish and whiten the teeth
- Evaluate the bite to insure balance and comfort
- Assess the effectiveness of the bite guard
- Reduce sensitivity if noted
- Evaluate health of dental implants
- Apply medications if needed

## General Dentist's Role During Maintenance

Even though your general dentist will likely be kept up-to-date with your progress during maintenance and advised of any problems that need attention, he or she is still responsible for your overall dental health. At least annual examinations are required to evaluate for new or recurrent decay, replace missing fillings and worn crowns as well as an overall check-up of your mouth.

## Smoking Cessation Programs

Due to the universal acceptance of smoking's influence on poor oral health, you can be certain that when you are ready to stop smoking, your periodontist will be ready to help. This may be via a referral to an area smoking-cessation program or the periodontal office may have its own stop-smoking program.

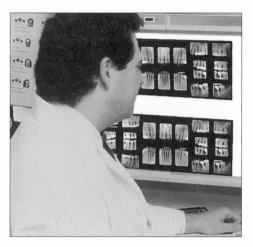

**Fig. 11-2**
Effective periodontal maintenance includes comparison of
x-rays and other clinical findings
over an extended period of time.
This type of monitoring can
insure the stabilty of the gums
and bone, as well as identify
early changes that may benefit
from attention.

## Periodic X-Rays

During the course of long term maintenance therapy, you can expect to have x-rays taken periodically to assess the bone stability around the teeth, development of dental decay and other abnormalities. Implants are usually x-rayed once during the first year, and depending on the situation, every one or two years thereafter.

## Maintenance...An Excellent Investment

Susceptible periodontal patients who are committed to a regular maintenance program will significantly reduce their chances of further gum disease. But even if there should be adverse changes in the health of their gums, the problems can be caught at an early stage when intervention is usually simple and predictable. And don't forget, early detection almost always means saving money.

A maintenance program, under the careful supervision of a periodontist, is probably as close as a patient can get to an insurance policy against advancing and recurrent periodontal disease. Once you start, stick to it. You will be glad you did!

# 12

# I'M GLAD YOU ASKED

## Questions Most Frequently Asked About Gum Disease and Dental Implants

### How much does periodontal (gum) treatment cost?

It's not facetious to say that the cost of periodontal therapy can range from ten dollars to between five and ten thousand dollars for all four quadrants of the mouth with comprehensive care including bone grafting and other advanced treatments. By investing in a good toothbrush and dental floss, a patient can reverse and cure the early stages of gum disease. The more sophisticated techniques required to treat advanced disease, demand greater skill and knowledge on the part of the specialist and therefore, a more significant investment.

### What about implant costs?

Remember that the implant procedure is usually comprised of separate stages. The first and second stages, performed by a periodontist, may incur a cost similar to a quadrant of periodontal surgery, plus the added expenditure for placing the implant, and any special associated procedures. The third stage is performed by your dentist and is similar to the cost of a non-implant supported prosthesis, in addition to the cost and preparation of the connections from the implant to the prosthesis.

### I have dental insurance, will it help pay for my treatment ?

There are many different insurance plans providing a wide range of dental benefits, some of which include periodontics and dental implants. In general, a request for a "pre-determination of benefits" of the anticipated treatment is sent to the insurance company, in order to ascertain the amount of assistance you can expect to receive.

### Can I catch gum disease from someone else?

According to a recent article in the *Journal of the American Dental Association*, family members or those in otherwise close contact, may be at risk for contracting periodontal disease. The research suggests that the disease-causing bacteria can be transferred in the saliva from parents to children and between couples.

### Is periodontal (gum) disease hereditary?

A predisposition or susceptibility to gum disease may be inherited. That is, if your parents or grandparents lost their teeth due to periodontal disease, a sensitivity to plaque that may result in periodontal disease could be passed on to their offspring.

The presence of genetic testing now makes it possible to identify certain patients with increased susceptibility. However, even with a predisposition to periodontal disease, a highly motivated patient who observes daily rigorous plaque control can usually ward off the loss of teeth.

### Does periodontal treatment or implant placement hurt ?

The answer to this question depends on the patient's threshold of pain and the therapist's skill. Use of appropriate instruments will reduce discomfort during scaling and root planing procedures. Periodontal surgery and implant placement are performed under local anesthesia, and therefore should be painless. Afterwards, proper use of post-operative medication and adherence to the periodontist's recommendations will reduce the likelihood of post-treatment problems.

In any surgical procedure, it is important that the patients consult with their therapist at the first hint of any problems or concern. An early call can lead to a speedy solution and avoid unnecessary discomfort.

## If I have periodontal disease...am I likely to develop a lot of decay?

The bacteria that cause periodontal diseases are generally different from those which cause decay. Therefore, it is possible for a patient to have a mouth free of decay or fillings and still have advanced periodontal disease. The opposite is also true. Patients with numerous fillings and new decay at every office visit frequently demonstrate no evidence of gum disease or bone loss.

Unfortunately, many patients tend to regard the lack of "cavities" as a general statement that their mouth is in top shape. This of course cannot be assumed, periodontal disease and dental decay are two different problems.

## How long does it take to complete treatment?

Generally, patients with early gingivitis will require several visits over the course of a month to return their mouth to a healthy state. If the problems are more advanced, a complete series of periodontal treatments including surgery, could take from three to six months or longer. The severity of the periodontal disease and approach to surgery (i.e. treating smaller or larger segments at each visit) will be a major factor influencing the duration of treatment.

Most implants require a waiting period of three to six months after surgical insertion before placement of the implant-supported prosthesis (tooth, bridge or denture).

## Is periodontal disease really preventable?

Yes, it is! There is no question that in the overwhelming majority of cases, if disease-free individuals are taught how to use dental floss and to brush their teeth properly – and continue to do so, they can expect to keep their teeth for the rest of their lives. In particular, the instruction of children at the earliest possible age will likely insure a healthy mouth through their adult years.

## What about a second opinion?

Patients who, after talking with their therapist, are uncertain about a recommendation regarding treatment, should most definitely seek a second opinion. Often the second opinion is sought after patients have been told that "everything is O.K.," despite the feeling that something seems wrong with their mouth. Patients may feel uneasy about asking for a second opinion for fear that their dentist will be insulted or resentful. There is no cause to be concerned. An ethical professional would not hesitate to cooperate with a patient who wishes to seek another opinion.

All specialists are accustomed to giving second opinions. This is neither good or bad. It's a phenomenon of life. A second opinion may give the patient another point of view or simply confirm the first recommendation, providing the extra level of confidence needed to begin therapy.

## My dental floss gets caught between my teeth! What's wrong?

Many patients complain that their floss doesn't pass easily between teeth, especially back ones. Usually the cause is fillings with uneven edges known as overhangs (Fig. 6-5). This can occur when fillings have cracked or frayed leaving irregular surfaces. Catches can also occur around crowns (caps) whose margins do not precisely fit the tooth.

All areas where dental floss does not pass smoothly along the teeth, are niches for bacterial plaque to colonize. The defective fillings or crowns should be repaired or replaced.

## Can't antibiotics be used instead of other kinds of treatment?

Antibiotics, both systemic and local, may be utilized as *adjunctive* therapy in certain forms of periodontal disease. Antibiotics may also be prescribed after surgery for a short period. However, routine use of long-term (potentially life saving) antibiotics as a stand-alone treatment is neither recommended nor effective.

## Who should perform periodontal and implant therapy?

Today, all dental schools teach diagnosis of periodontal diseases and their treatment in the early, uncomplicated stages, as well as the basic principles of dental implants.

Therefore, a patient can expect that their family dentist may be the first to recognize and sometimes treat gum disease at its earliest stages. If the progress of the disease is more advanced or associated with complicating factors, consultation with a periodontal specialist is a good idea. Regarding implant therapy, the team approach (page 101) has the advantage of providing the best combination of skill and experience.

## Are implants sometimes sensitive to cold or hot like natural teeth?

No. While in every other respect dental implants may feel just like your own teeth, unlike natural teeth there are no nerves running through the implant, so there is no temperature sensitivity.

## Can lasers be used for gum surgery?

Today, the only approved function for lasers by the FDA (Federal Drug Administration) in periodontics is for soft tissue surgery, such as gingivectomy. However, the high cost of the equipment, its restricted indications and the need for special safeguards have limited its use in periodontal surgery. The field of medical lasers does have great potential. With increased application and proven benefits, a more significant role for this tool in periodontal surgery can be expected.

## What about seeing my family dentist?

You probably have a family or general dentist who is being kept up-to-date with your treatment through correspondence from the periodontist's office. The two professionals work together to insure you receive all the required treatment in a timely and coordinated fashion throughout the course of therapy. Your periodontist may consult with the dentist regarding changing fillings, new crowns or other restorations, especially in areas of plaque and food catches. After periodontal treatment, you will probably continue to see your periodontist for maintenance, and your dentist for all your other dental needs, including at least a yearly check up.

# PART IV

---

## *Appendix*

# RESOURCES

The following resources have been compiled for the reader who would like to enhance his/her knowledge of dentistry in general, the specialty of periodontics as well as access to institutions and health care providers in the profession.

**THE AMERICAN DENTAL ASSOCIATION (ADA)**
For general information on dentistry and related subjects in the United States:
211 East Chicago Avenue
Chicago, IL 60611
Tel: (312) 440-2500
Web site: http://www.ada.org

**THE CANADIAN DENTAL ASSOCIATION (CDA)**
For general information on dentistry and related subjects in Canada:
1815 Alta Vista
Ottawa (Ontario)
K1G3Y6
Tel: (613) 523-1770
Web site: http://www.cda-ada.ca

**THE AMERICAN ACADEMY OF PERIODONTOLOGY (AAP)**
For information on periodontists, periodontics and dental implants.
The Academy also provides a free referral service to a periodontist in your area.
Suite 800
737 N. Michigan Avenue
Chicago IL 60611-2690.
Tel: (312) 787-3670
Web site: http://www.perio.org

**INSTITUTIONS WITH POST GRADUATE PROGRAMS IN PERIODONTICS**
If you still have difficulty finding either a periodontist or information regarding periodontics or dental implants, try contacting the following institutions. They have ADA approved programs which train specialists in periodontics, and may be able to provide additional assistance.

**ALABAMA**
University of Alabama
School of Dentistry
Birmingham    (205) 934-5426

**CALIFORNIA**
University of California, LA
UCLA School of Dentistry
Los Angeles    (310) 825-5543

Veterans Administration Medical Center
Dental Service 691/W160
Los Angeles    (310) 824-3202

University of California, SF
Department of Stomatology
San Francisco    (415) 476-8958

Loma Linda University
School of Dentistry
Loma Linda    (909) 824-4610

University of Southern California
School of Dentistry
Los Angeles    (213) 740-2841

**CONNECTICUT**
University of Connecticut
School of Dental Medicine
Farmington    (203) 679-2383

**FLORIDA**
Nova Southeastern University
College of Dental Medicine
Ft. Lauderdale    (954) 262-1613

University of Florida
College of Dentistry
Gainesville    (904) 392-4305

**GEORGIA**
Medical College of Georgia
School of Dentistry
Augusta    (706) 721-2441

**ILLINOIS**
University of Illinois at Chicago
College of Dentistry
Chicago    (312) 413-8405

Northwestern University Dental School
Chicago    (312) 503-7809

**INDIANA**
Indiana University
School of Dentistry
Indianapolis    (317) 274-4468

Indianapolis Veterans Medical Center
Medical Center Dental Service
Indianapolis    (317) 267-8733

**IOWA**
The University of Iowa
College of Dentistry
Iowa City    (319) 335-7238

**KENTUCKY**
University of Kentucky
School of Dentistry
Lexington    (606) 233-6250

University of Louisville
School of Dentistry
Louisville    (502) 852-5086

**LOUISIANA**
Louisiana State University
School of Dentistry
New Orleans    (504) 619-8610

**MARYLAND**
Baltimore College of Dental Surgery
Baltimore    (410) 706-7152

**MASSACHUSETTS**
Boston University
Goldman School of Graduate Dentistry
Boston    (617) 638-4762

Harvard School of Dental Medicine
Boston    (617) 432-1452

Tufts University
School of Dental Medicine
Boston    (617) 936-6532

**MICHIGAN**
The University of Michigan
School of Dentistry
Ann Arbor    (313) 764-9148

**MINNESOTA**
Mayo Graduate School of Medicine
Rochester    (507) 284-8410

University of Minnesota
College of Dentistry
Minneapolis    (612) 625-9107

Indianapolis Veterans Medical Center
Medical Center Dental Service
Indianapolis    (317) 267-8733

**MISSOURI**
University of Missouri-Kansas
School of Dentistry
Kansas City    (816) 235-5210

Saint Louis University
School of Dentistry
St. Louis    (314) 977-2240

**NEBRASKA**
University of Nebraska Medical Center
Lincoln    (402) 472-1273

**NEW JERSEY**
New Jersey University School of
Medicine and Dentistry
Newark    (201) 982-4210

**NEW YORK**
Columbia University
School of Dental and Oral Surgery
New York    (212) 305-9292

Veterans Administration Medical Center
New York    (212) 686-7500

Eastman Dental Center
Rochester    (816) 275-5046

New York University
College of Dentistry
New York    (212) 998-9735

State University of New York at Buffalo
School of Dental Medicine
Buffalo    (716) 831-3940

State University of New York
at Stony Brook
School of Dental Medicine
Stony Brook    (516) 632-8895

**NORTH CAROLINA**
University of North Carolina
School of Dentistry
Chapel Hill    (919) 966-2701

**OHIO**
Case Western Reserve University
School of Dentistry
Cleveland    (216) 368-3277

Ohio State University
College of Dentistry
Columbus    (614) 292-2218

**OKLAHOMA**
University of Oklahoma
College of Dentistry
Oklahoma City    (405) 271-6531

**OREGON**
Oregon Health Sciences University
School of Dentistry
Portland    (503) 494-8874

**PENNSYLVANIA**
University of Pennsylvania
School of Dental Medicine
Philadelphia    (215) 898-3268

University of Pittsburgh
School of Dental Medicine
Pittsburgh    (412) 648-8602

Temple University
School of Dentistry
Philadelphia    (215) 221-2926

**INSTITUTIONS WITH POST GRADUATE PROGRAMS IN PERIODONTICS (continued...)**

**SOUTH CAROLINA**
Medical University of South Carolina
College of Dental Medicine
Charleston    (803) 792-3907

**TENNESSEE**
University of Tennessee, Memphis
Memphis    (901) 448-6242

**TEXAS**
Texas A&M Univ. System
Dallas    (214) 828-8126

University of Texas Health Science Center
At Houston/Dental Branch
Houston    (713) 792-4047

University of Texas Health Science
Center at San Antonio
San Antonio    (210) 567-3600

**VIRGINIA**
Virginia Commonwealth University
School of Dentistry
Richmond    (804) 786-0786

**WASHINGTON**
University of Washington
School of Dentistry
Seattle    (206) 543-1568

**WISCONSIN**
Zablocki Veterans Administration
Medical Center
Dental Clinic/160
Milwaukee    (414) 384-2000

**CANADA**

**BRITISH COLUMBIA**
The University of British Columbia
Faculty of Dentistry
Vancouver    (604) 822-6822

**MANITOBA**
The University of Manitoba
Faculty of Dentistry
Winnipeg    (204) 7878-6597

**NOVA SCOTIA**
Dalhousie University
Faculty of Dentistry
Halifax    (902) 494-1419

**ONTARIO**
University of Ontario
Faculty of Dentistry
Toronto    (416) 979-4408

# INDEX

*Few gifts are as valued as the gift of a beautiful, natural looking smile.*

THE THIRD, FULLY REVISED EDITION OF
**IGNORE YOUR TEETH and THEY'LL GO AWAY**
**The Complete Guide To Gum Disease**
By Periodontist, Sheldon D. Sydney, D.D.S.

Please send me ___copies of **IGNORE YOUR TEETH and THEY'LL GO AWAY**

@ a cost of (# Books x 28$)_____

Shipping and handling $8.95 ($13.95 outside U.S.) per copy_____

Maryland and Canadian residents add sales tax_____

Total enclosed or charge to credit card_____

Send to:

Name _____

Address _____

City _____State_____ Zip code_____

Country (if outside the U.S.) _____

❏ Check enclosed

❏ Charge my credit card, check one:

      ❏ Visa   ❏ Mastercard

      card #_____ expiration date_____

Signature:_____

**Mail or fax completed form to:**      **or e-mail to:**

Book Sales      booksales@devida.com

Devida Publications

205 John Eager Court

Pikesville Maryland 21208

Fax: 410-484-4802

# About the Author

Dr. Sheldon Dov Sydney is a Diplomate of the American Board of Periodontology and Clinical Associate Professor of Periodontics at The University of Maryland School of Dentistry, the first dental college in the world. He is also on the faculty of the Postgraduate Program in Periodontics at Tel Aviv University, Israel and formerly clinical instructor in Periodontics at Emory University, Georgia. In addition to authoring three editions of this consumer's guide, Dr. Sydney has published scientific articles in the profession's leading journals. He is a member of the American Academy of Periodontology and has been honored with Fellowships in both the American and International Colleges of Dentists. He served as President of the Maryland Association of Periodontists and Associate Editor, Journal of the Maryland State Dental Association.

Besides writing and teaching, Dr. Sydney maintains a full-time private practice limited to periodontics and dental implants.